6 Steps to Health & Happiness

A simple and easy to follow guide to
combining physical health and a good
mental attitude to reach true health
and lasting happiness.

ARUNYA VILLIERS

The contents of this book are based upon the experience of the author and presented for educational purposes only. The information in this book is not intended to diagnose or prescribe for medical or psychological conditions, nor to recommend specific information, products or services as treatment of disease or to provide diagnosis. The information contained herein is not intended to replace a relationship with a doctor or a qualified health care professional. The reader should be aware that this information is not intended as medical advice, but rather a sharing of knowledge and the results may vary depending upon use and commitment. The author encourages you to make your own health care decisions based upon your research and in partnership with a qualified health care professional.

www.ArunyaVilliers.com

Printed in the United States of America.

ISBN: 978-1-312-97843-0

I dedicate this book to YOU, my reader, in the hopes that you can begin a new life today and truly become healthy and happy. I thank everyone who has been by my side through my journeys as well as those who have taught me the important lessons in life without which I would not be where I am today.

CONTENTS

PREFACE

Why you are here

I've written this book to help people from all walks of life, no matter the age, situation or health level to achieve the main thing we all search and long for, true happiness. And to find true happiness, it's essential that we are healthy as you cannot be happy if you are feeling sick or struggling with an illness. No matter where you currently find yourself or what struggles you are facing, I'm sure you agree that at the end of the day you just want to be happy. I'm genuinely passionate about getting as many people to this perfect and balanced state not just because I love the idea of everyone being healthy but also because I'm incredibly passionate about the planet and the choices that make you healthy will also inevitably help the environment around you. Of course my main focus is to get people healthy through holistic and nutritional coaching but my passion spreads much further than that. The same things that harm you and plague your sickness also poisons the planet so hence my reasoning for wanting to reach as many people as possible with this. I'm very concerned with the environment, the global warming, the polluted oceans, the effects of our consumer lifestyle on the planet, the loss of natural habitats, growing list of extinct animals and many other issues, which are all tied in with this 6 step program to get you healthy. I believe that a society that is happier overall will benefit everyone and make life in general a more positive and beautiful experience. That is truly my wish for the world.

I have read so many books on every topic of health, heard a variety of discussions, watched all the documentaries, read numerous blogs and articles, seen the programs and shows over the years and have always wondered why the physical health and enlightenment guides to happiness are so separate instead of being worked on in unison. I don't think one can exist without the other and to me both are equally as important. A happy mind and a healthy body go hand in hand and if you don't have the balance of both then there is no way to truly reach the full potential of what you can be. Let me explain further what I really mean about the physical and mental functioning in balance.

I have clients who come to me and say, 'I decided to get healthy and I've done everything I can think of. I eat really well, I've removed toxins from my food and diet, I exercise like a madman, I have cut all the junk food and unhealthy things that don't serve my body well, I read all the labels at the grocery store and avoid anything that's unnatural but I'm still suffering. My body is not functioning well, I'm constantly aching, I can't sleep well, I'm getting sick all the time and I feel depressed. Am I missing something?' and that's when I know that they don't have a good balance between a healthy body and a healthy mind. They worked really hard at the physical aspect of things but ignored the mental aspect and with the mental aspect being ignored, it will literally make you physically unwell. I will ask them questions like, 'Have you eliminated stress from your life? What is your favorite pastime? Do you meditate? What is it that you love most about yourself? How often do you spend time in nature or outdoors? What good do you do for the community? Do you experience anxiety daily? Are your relationships with others healthy?' and they are often confused by this questioning and wonder what it has to do with their health but in reality it has everything to do with their health. Choosing to become 100% physically healthy but ignoring your mental state will not get you the results you are looking for because no matter how well you eat and how much you exercise, if you are living with chronic stress, functioning as a workaholic, not managing your anxiety, giving no time to love yourself or do enjoyable activities and in a habit of constant negative thinking, it will affect every cell and organ in your body eventually causing illness and disease.

Then there is the other side of the extreme where someone has done everything to become a really good person but yet they ignore their own physical needs. They have read every book on enlightenment, are immensely spiritual, meditate daily, practice good deeds, live their passion, have given themselves to a higher purpose and constantly give to others but they struggle as their health isn't great which leads to feeling unwell mentally and eventually they get beat down, tired and are left exhausted. So although they have excelled at living in the most positive way mentally, they have failed to truly take care of themselves at the physical level and without that there is no way you can feel good.

This program I wrote addresses the TWO main elements that a human being needs to feel good. Part one is to fix all the physical issues so that your body can be fully healthy and part two is addressing all the mental aspects to change the habits that will affect your life in a positive and fruitful way instead of damaging it. I also wanted to focus on writing something that would be simple and easy to follow. I want the reader to be able to read each chapter and immediately change their lifestyle with the exercises that follow without the chapter going into lengthy explanations or the history of each topic.

The PHYSICAL ELEMENT:

When you are toxic and deficient in numerous nutrients, suffering on a physical level, there is no way that the rest of you can function well. When you have bad habits, for years of over eating, eating low quality junk food, drinking alcohol or smoking, taking numerous pills or drugs and poisoning yourself with artificial and chemical additives, your brain is 100% fully toxic. Everything you ingest is absorbed and stored in your body in small amounts that keep adding up over time. So your brain that was perfectly healthy at birth is now filled with tiny deposits of poisons (I'm just speaking of the brain in this example but this is happening to all your organs). So you have a brain that is under incredible strain as it's still trying to function although it's so much more difficult than it should be. Now on top of putting in poisons and toxins into your body, you are also eating low grade food that doesn't have the nutritional content it should, so you're not only poisoning but you are also depleting your body of nutrients that it needs. Just like a car that has to have oil, gas, water to function, your body is a complex creation that needs every single nutrient that it was designed to receive. Your brain requires numerous things to function properly, for example if you take out one vital thing from your diet like the omega 3 fatty acid that helps your brain in the cognitive processes which controls all the information that enters your brain, without which you cannot function at your peak. Suddenly taking in information becomes hard, focusing becomes impossible, the attention span is low, logic and reasoning are out the window, long and short term memory suffers and so on and so on. Of course that's an example of only one item that I discussed while our brains also require the vitamin B family, zinc, protein, vitamin C, vitamin D, vitamin E, carbohydrates, calcium. So after years and years of pumping toxins into the brain as well as making it highly nutrient deficient, I'm surprised that people still function as well as they do and this abusive cycle affects you and your life so directly that you can't imagine. Over the years you become chronically sad, tired, unmotivated, sickly, confused, depressed, constantly in aches and pains, unhappy and it seems that everything in your life is suffering and that things aren't going your way. A lot of the time it's really about what's happening in your body on a physical level that's the root of the problem because without good health you cannot begin to work on the mental issues. So many people jump from this diet to that diet, read this book and run off to that lecture, then they try that life changing weekend course with their friend and then go to the new yoga studio for a month and then listen to the 'fix your life' audio books but wonder why none of it worked. Well it's because there is a method that must be followed. You cannot think clearly or focus on the changes you want to make in your life if your physical body isn't healthy, so now you know why that should always be the first step. You want to do better at work, push harder at your goals, have more fulfilling relationships, feel great, have more energy and so forth but first, you must address the physical state of your body.

The MENTAL ELEMENT:

The second part of the program consists of removing the toxic behavioral patterns and negative thinking to achieve a perfect state of mind that doesn't constantly harm us and instead improves our physical and mental state. It then helps us to be able to bring in the positivity through reminding us what we enjoy and show us how to enjoy it. Just like the first part, it's very important as you can be the most physically healthy person in the world but if you can't take the next step and eliminate bad habits, negative thoughts, damaging behavior, chronic stress, constant judgment of others, constant critique of yourself, poisonous vocal and physical actions then you will not find happiness. Science has proven what many thought for decades, that your mental attitude, thoughts and behavior directly affect your physical body and that a lot of disease is also caused by what's happening on a mental level. The energy you feel or carry around with you is affecting every single cell in your body and everything is connected, it's all a circle of life and you can't just choose one single element to fix or master but must address the entire phenomenon of your being. Currently the rate of depression is at it's peak and people are doing everything they can to avoid, cure, fix or eliminate this disease that plagues the mind cutting off motivation to do anything. It ruins life every single day often leading to months or years of lost time and makes every relationship of the depressed individual suffer. Not only do relationships suffer but everything falls apart including work, career, families, pretty much every aspect is affected when you live for an extended period of time with depression. Maybe the depressed person tries to get help eventually but that just leads to being sent back and forth between psychologists and psychiatrists, doing numerous lengthy and expensive therapy sessions, ordering tests, then being pumped with toxic pills and drugs that promise to balance the chemicals in the brain and stabilize the moods but instead it just further confuses the body and mind with more toxins without much relief, eventually leaving the person in a zombie-like state which makes it even more impossible to see a way out. And depression has become a normal occurrence with everyone accepting that it just happens and the medical community doesn't offer much hope in terms of a cure. Pretty much everyone has been affected by it or knows someone who has depression and it seems to be such a hopeless scenario yet in my opinion it's just a symptom of a body that's out of balance and not being cared for on the physical and mental level.

In my opinion all disease, whether it's physical or mental, is never caused by one single variable but a collection of causes that are both external like toxins, incorrect food, bad air quality as well as internal like chronic stress, negative thinking, anxiety and so on. All of these causes collect and build up over time and you don't just get sick overnight but it's a slow and almost unnoticeable decline of health. You have less and less energy, you get certain symptoms, constant pains and aches, you think foggy, you see blurry, you eventually don't have much motivation to do anything, you are constantly exhausted and sleeping unwell and your mental state seems to be in a fog without ever feeling clear or awake. You eventually go to your doctor because you don't feel good and the doctor will prescribe you drugs that only cover up the symptoms temporarily or order more tests that are harmful. Never do you wake up having more energy or feel great again but what you do experience is this downward spiral on all levels and most people usually accept this as normal and attest it to just simply 'getting older'. And you take more and more pills and treatments prescribed to address the symptoms you are experiencing but the cause is hardly ever looked at and it's almost like you're playing a cat and mouse game with your health in a never ending cycle as whatever pills you are taking for this symptom will inevitably cause another pain or issue with your health and then you take a new pill to cover that symptom and so on.

I believe this way of functioning is not only harmful physically as you're putting your body through so much torment but it's also counter productive and it makes you really exhausted. I'm sure we can all agree that if you are incorrectly feeding your body, living with chronic stress, eating poisons and chemicals, functioning with anxiety and all the other debilitating life choices that go into an unhealthy lifestyle, that eventually we should expect to fall ill. And why wouldn't our mental state be affected by this as well? Depression and any other mental illness is greatly affected by our lifestyle choices with scientific evidence showing that food, exercise, sunlight, etc, directly affects our brain function and mood. Evidence also shows that our mental attitude, our energy and thoughts directly affects us on a physical level. You must be ready to address both your physical body and your mind if you want to be healthy and you also must be ready to address both to reach happiness as addressing one and ignoring the other will give you no good result. Our bodies were designed to function in harmony and balance as nature intended and every single part and cell of our bodies is connected. Finding that harmony and balance isn't as impossible as one might think and once you do, you will be amazed as to how easily and quickly all your issues melt away no matter if they are physical or mental.

Now just like it's taken a lot of variables and a lot of time to cause whatever illness or issue you're battling with, most of us battling with numerous issues at any given time, it also takes time, consistency and work to reverse all the damage. You can't fix any one illness, disease or problem in your life by just changing one thing. There is no magic pill or an overnight cure that can reverse all the negative choices that were made over the years so if you keep looking for that quick fix, you will be disappointed. You have to commit to the process from beginning to end so that you can begin to enjoy life again. You will need to eliminate all the causes of suffering by going through all the steps that address your physical and mental states. The true beauty of when you follow the steps one by one is that you are not targeting just one illness, just one symptom, just one issue, but you will eliminate all the issues at once, no matter what they might be. This is about bringing your body and mind to the purest form it can possibly be at and although it might not be possible for you to do everything at once, or maybe it won't be possible for you to do it as fast as you'd like, this is your guidebook and a starting point so you can get yourself on track starting now. I believe that most problems you have in your life will be either completely eliminated or at the very least very much improved by following this. Whether you are chronically vexed with tumors, constantly debilitated by illnesses, just feeling horrible for no reason, have issues with your relationships, never have energy, feel lost in life or have mental instabilities, these issues all stem from the same cause of your body being out of balance. The beauty in all of these steps is that not only is it great for you, but every one of these steps is in turn helping the environment and the planet because if we live in harmony and balance with our bodies, then we are also living in harmony and balance with the world around us.

So being healthy physically and being healthy mentally must both be mastered and they must be addressed in the correct order otherwise you will be faced with an impossible challenge and you will spend the rest of your life trying to figure out a riddle with no solution.

I think it's time for a wake up call as our world is in peril on every level, environmentalists keep sending us warning signals that things aren't looking good, we are seeing what used to be rare and horrific diseases emerge in younger and younger kids, mental illness is on the rise pretty much affecting every single person and obesity is growing at an alarming rate. It's not that people are ignorant to everything that's happening around them but it's the result of being so sickly and so exhausted that they don't have energy for anything except trying to make it through their day. Most people are struggling with either trying pull through financially or surviving emotionally. Most are constantly living in pain, waiting for that day when everything might be better, living as if life is a jail sentence, not living as we should. How many of us feel that most of the time we are functioning at 10% of our capacity? Why can't we function at a 100% all the time?

No matter where you live in the world, you can look around and see everyone scrambling along the sidewalk, rushing with their cellphone in one hand and bag in the other, running to their meeting, job, gym, lunch, school. Most people's faces clearly tell you they are sad, riddled with problems. Why do most people feel so unsatisfied with their lives? And were we ever happier than we are now? Technological advances are plenty, we have more comforts than any generation before us, most of the world isn't plagued by war and a huge percentage of us have a roof over our head and enough food to survive. I don't believe we were designed to live a life of misery nor do I think we were designed to always want more and more. I don't know if our true nature was to be negative, short tempered, selfish and unkind and if asked about happiness, I'm sure everyone would say they wish to be happy, so what's stopping us from overcoming that barrier and reaching our potential? Is it the lack of knowledge? Is it the lack of motivation? Is it the toxic food that we've been eating for an extended period of time? Is it being stuck in our old patterns and habits? I sometimes wonder if the way things used to be long long ago was actually better for us?

Long ago there were no processed foods and you didn't have to struggle to get a job, work long hours, or struggle to get by. You didn't go hungry when the next person over had tons of food, you didn't have bills, have a car to drive, nor did you live in isolation but instead you lived in a community or tribe. Nobody took more than they needed and hoarding food or possessions was seen as a mental illness. People ate food that was local and in season that was nutritious, fresh and non toxic. Humans didn't over eat, they didn't eat abnormal amounts of sugar and they didn't' eat while staring at the TV. There was no GMO's, no quick cook meals, no cereals, no microwave foods, no meats filled with hormones or meal replacement shakes. The air was clean and they didn't take pills of any kind and medicinal herbs were used in moderation. It wasn't standard to have 10 surgeries by the time you reached the age of 60 and you didn't spend your time on laptops, Ipads, Iphones or kindles. Humans made eye contact regularly and had genuine relationships that included vocal and physical exchange on a constant basis filling the need for true human connection. They didn't multitask to save time nor did they live in severely overpopulated areas where you didn't have the necessary space to feel sane. They lived closer to nature and they lived with nature, not separating themselves from the earth with floors, walls, ceilings and roofs, getting to gaze at the sky or lay in the green lush all day long. They also didn't spend all their time sitting... sitting all day at the computer, at work, indoors, away from the sunlight, away from nature and all things that are truly important to your well being. Humans back then spent their time running, swimming, walking, playing, dancing, singing, eating... There was no stress induced by errands, phone calls, banks, taxes, bills, insurance. They were able to connect to their children and spend real quality time with them every day as there were no time constraints. They were able to enjoy every single thing they did as there was no rush, no obligation, no pressure.

Currently we have all the technology we can imagine which obviously makes our lives easier and simpler and we can do things so much faster. We have the comforts of everything that a modern civilized society can offer and of course it's nice that we don't have to wash our clothing in the river and that we can share photos to everyone in the world at the click of a mouse... we gained so much in comparison of what we gave up. Or did we? Nobody is saying that we should be living in the woods like cave men but maybe we can figure out how to take all the comforts and appreciate them without going overboard, without becoming dependent on them and without being able to find time for things that are truly important. After all, the technological advances are there so we can do things faster and with more ease so why do we now have less time for things we enjoy then we ever did? I think it's time to remember what's truly important in life and find balance. Although we have spent decades evolving and growing in many areas, we definitely have gotten worse at enjoying simple pleasures and being in the moment. It doesn't seem that many things bring us happiness or the happiness is very short lived yet we don't stop accumulating material possessions, stop yearning to have more wealth, wishing for more success and more recognition. There is this sickening need to be wealthy, to be so rich, to not be ordinary, to be recognized, to not be a failure. We want so much to be better, we need to be better... better than who? Better than your neighbor? Your brother? Your best friend?

Part of the work is becoming awake and I'm speaking of an awakening that allows us to not only evolve on a technological level, an educational level, a scientific level or being stronger, faster, living longer but to start evolving mentally too. Imagine a world where everyone was constantly aware of each and every moment. Imagine a world where every bite of food consumed would taste amazing and would bring magical healing and nutrition to our bodies. Imagine a world where nobody was out of touch, nobody was selfish, nobody lost their temper or hurt one another. Imagine a world where disease didn't exist and where everyone lived in harmony with each other and the planet. Imagine a world where every single person felt happy and fulfilled. Maybe this sounds like total fiction but maybe it's possible for us all to work towards that?

You might be wondering why I'm speaking about all these matters. Maybe you bought this book to lose weight or to get healthy and you're confused why you're reading about peace on our planet and being the happiest you can be. You might be wondering why we are not talking about cleansing and juicing. You might even be frustrated and wish to skip to the next chapter but I hope you don't as I really need you to understand how everything goes hand in hand and why I don't feel that it's possible for health and happiness to exist without each other.

The program that I have created will certainly work for anyone who is willing to commit without picking and choosing certain parts but doing it all correctly step by step from beginning to end. I can guarantee you that you will come out a healthier and happier person at the other end of this book if you take part at 100% of your ability. Every chapter has exercises at the end of it and before you move onto the next chapter it's vital that you complete all of the exercises of the chapter you just read. Do not rush through it and do the exercises efficiently and fully. Depending on your schedule, it's okay to spread the exercises over a couple or more days. If you are really busy one day and can't do much that's okay, just do it the next day but make a decision on whether you're serious about this and don't skip more than a couple of days during this process. If you do fall behind and start skipping days without doing then work then you will be sending yourself the message that your health and happiness isn't that important to you. You want to trust yourself and so you can't be the person who lets yourself down. Nobody will make the changes for you that you need to make and nobody can magically fix everything without you doing the work. It's time to put an end to being the person who can never commit to anything or being the person who never completes anything. It's important that we give this a proper chance and fight off the urge to make excuses or to procrastinate. This is your life and you need to make a decision now that enough is enough and you are tired of being sick, being unhealthy and being emotionally and physically exhausted. I can honestly promise you that if you are willing, this will change your life. This guide is a great tool to address all your issues and it's easy to read with no big words or lengthy historical explanations that you can't understand. Some chapters will be longer and more in depth and others will be shorter. Some chapters will be followed by a lot of exercises and some will have a few. Some exercises will require lots of writing, keeping track and home work, but make sure to do them and don't get lazy. Don't think that you can just make notes in your head as that's not as effective so when asked to write something down, actually write it down. I recommend getting a notebook specifically for this work and make this a project that you work on with dedication and excitement.

STEP ONE

Eliminate the poisons

When we are born we are as perfect as we will ever be but unfortunately that's precisely the moment when we start collecting toxins in our bodies and research now shows that toxins begin accumulating long before we are born, while we are still in the womb. From the polluted air to the chemically enhanced food, every minute is filled with our bodies absorbing poisons through our mouth, skin and the air. The body constantly tries to flush out the toxins but with the chemicals being so many and the amounts of them being so high, the body struggles to keep up. Inevitably after years of abuse and a toxin saturated environment, our bodies are no longer able to flush out the toxins thoroughly or fast enough and your body crosses the line where it is accumulating more toxins than it can expel. This is when the toxins in your body start to build up and be stored, and they are stored everywhere! They build up in our brain, organs, lungs, intestines, glands and although eating healthier and improving your lifestyle helps, if you don't minimize your exposure to toxins and eliminate them from your home and life then you'll never catch up in the clean up process. Before can begin detoxing, you need to make sure that you thoroughly go through all the ways you can make your life cleaner. You can't control all of your environments and variables but there is a lot that you can control and everything needs to be looked at from your workplace to your dinner table to your home. A lot of this chapter will be about replacing many items you use on a daily basis with a more natural alternative that might be more expensive but just remember that nothing is more important than your health so avoid saving money now to not get sick later. Of course you cannot completely rid your life of toxins and not everyone can eliminate everything I speak about in this chapter but the more you can say goodbye to, the better, so take charge and clean it up!

THE HOME:

Our home, it's the place where we spend most of our time and the place that's meant to be safe and protected yet it's covered from floor to ceiling in toxins. People spend so much time to choose a neighborhood that is safe, a place that looks nice, a home that has a great view and so many other wise decisions to keep themselves and their family happy and free from harm but then they go out and purchase countless toxic products that they bring home and spread to each and every room. Your children spend all their time at that house, growing up, while playing on the carpet and crawling around on the ground, which is of course laden with chemicals. And it's not only the carpet or the floor but the windows, toilet bowls, counters, dishes, clothing and so on. Most people don't realize that pretty much every inch of their home is spreading some sort of toxin that will be breathed in, absorbed by the skin or put into the mouth. This is a scary thought and if you have children even scarier so don't Eliminating as many toxins and poisons as you can in your home is vital and probably the easiest of the changes. We spend a lot of time in our home and although cleaning up toxins at work helps too it's the home where we have the most control as to what we want to bring inside. Don't put a price tag on your health and don't hold onto anything for any reason, just remember you are doing it for the health of you and your family.

Household cleaners

These are some of the most toxic and unnecessary things found in most homes. I can promise you that there is hardly anything you cannot clean with either baking soda, vinegar or lemon juice. They all have their own specific whitening, anti grease and anti bacterial properties and with either one or the combination of all of them you can take on any cleaning duties. After using them you will see that you have no reason to be using toxic chemicals in your home where you eat, sleep and spend most of your time. Not only is it toxic for you but it's toxic for your pets, family and the environment. Pouring bleach down your drain is a horrible idea if you take a second to think about where it goes. None of the cleaning solutions require any mandatory testing for safety on humans and the fumes alone can be incredibly harmful. We assume that these products must be safe to use since we purchased them at a store but this is a huge mistake. Throw away all your laundry detergent, dish washing liquids, carpet shampoos, toilet cleaners, window cleaners, bleach, floor and tile cleaners, bathtub cleaners and anything else that isn't natural and commit to natural cleaning solutions. People are so obsessed with having a cleaning liquid for every surface and purpose which is so unnecessary. Often parents clean even more religiously when they have children running around but research shows that kids who grow up in incredibly sterile homes actually have weaker immune systems and are prone to get sick much more often so do away with all these toxic cleaners in your home. Every single cleaning solution you look at will have hazard and warnings at the back of the bottle, why do you want these in your home?

I have included recipes in the last chapter for your all the cleaning solutions you might need. You can make these in bulk amounts and also save money in addition to saving your health. If you cannot make your own and must buy your cleaning solutions then make sure to buy the non toxic, environmentally friendly cleaners even if they are a little more pricy. They now make everything in a natural option so there can be no more excuses.

Medications

As a society we are so used to taking a pill the second we feel anything unpleasant that we don't ever stop to think about whether it's really necessary. Pills are swallowed so carelessly and so often without any forethought. What does the medication you are taking have in it? How unnatural are the chemicals used in making the pill? What are the long term side effects of taking this? What damage is caused by just taking one of these? What about a hundred? What warnings does the insert include? The truth of the matter is that every time you consume a pill of any kind, you are poisoning yourself. Even if it's a tiny amount of poison each time, when you are doing this on a daily basis, constantly putting different drugs into your body, eventually it will take a toll. Making your body be a dumpster of cocktails of medications is never a good idea and tiny deposits of these medications will remain in your body and cause harm. Of course at times it is inevitable that you have to take medications, but make sure that it's an absolute necessity and that you have exhausted all the natural alternatives. There are hundreds of books available that offer so many natural remedies so why would you not choose to try those first? Initially when you feel ill, I would personally recommend to wait a minimum of 48 hours before even thinking about any sort of medication even if it's something as "innocent" as aspirin or ibuprofen. Often with some rest from solid food, plenty of water and a good amount of sleep, the condition is eliminated. You have to give your body a chance to fight off anything naturally whether it's a cold or a headache before you medicate yourself. If you are in severe pain then of course you won't be able to avoid taking painkillers but don't make it a habit to pop a pill at even the slightest headache. Getting a sore throat does not mean you need to drink flu pills, cough syrups and anti congestion medication in the first hour you feel it coming on. Instead try resting as well as gargling every 20 minutes with warm sea salt water. Forgo your medications for some herbal tea with honey and a teaspoon of food based vitamin C powder in a glass of water drank every hour. If you get a headache then try drinking a few glasses of water first as headaches are often a sign of dehydration. There are so many great alternative therapy health books on the market and with the internet you have numerous ideas at your fingertips to fix many issues. Especially when it comes to children, be weary of being too quick to offer them chemical solutions as their bodies are so much more sensitive. Becoming dependent on certain medications and taking them often results in a lifetime of damage to organs. Often times having the pills on hand makes it so much harder not to take it as soon as you have a headache or any other ache so I advise you now to go through them and throw out all those pills that are randomly stacked in your medicine cabinet. Throw out as many as you can if not all and make sure that the ones you do keep are really necessary as well as not expired.

Toiletries

A lot of you might not be able to part with your favorite shampoo, face cream or deodorant which is understandable but make sure you take the time to look into each and every product you use and commit to trying to find a natural alternative or if you can go without it. Of course it's not always possible for everyone to only use natural or home made toiletries, but keep in mind how counter productive it is to be eating right, getting healthy, exercising but then caking on pounds of toxic lip sticks, creams, shower gels and so on. It's a mistake when you only think about health when it comes to what you're eating as being healthy includes avoiding toxins and unnatural materials in all areas. You have to realize that anything you put onto your skin, even in tiny amounts, will be absorbed. Every item you use has hundreds of chemicals and think about how many products you use on your body per day? An average person easily uses over twenty products a day and with every one of those containing a cocktail of chemicals, how could that be good for a body? You have no more excuses as even if you don't have the time to make your own home make toiletries, most stores carry a huge selection of natural alternatives so to keep using things that harm you and complicate your health doesn't make sense. Often it will take some time to find the natural products that you like and that work for you but remember there cannot be compromises when it comes to your health, no color of lipstick is worth swallowing pounds of mercury so commit to only using natural products. Make sure you check all the ingredients on your toiletries you use now and immediately discard anything that isn't natural. Remember that using anything that's laden with chemicals will not only add to you being unhealthy but it will also speed up aging and cause skin damage. Also don't forget to avoid using sun screens that are not natural as those are known to actually cause cancer instead of prevent it. Use an all natural zinc oxide sun screen to protect yourself. Choose natural toothpaste without fluoride, use natural soap, natural make up and natural lotions (coconut oil is so good for your skin to moisturize and so much cheaper).

Microwave

THROW IT OUT! No matter if your microwave is more advanced and less harmful than the older models, it's still not worth it. Cooking something in a microwave that is meant to fuel your body and give it nutrition isn't right. You might argue that it's incredibly convenient but the convenience doesn't outweigh the dangers. Microwaved food has so many draw backs and keeps cooking long after you've eaten it, which is a scary reality. Anything you wish to warm up can be defrosted, warmed up or cooked on your stove top. Don't be temped by having it there, dispose of it as soon as you can.

<u>Cooking pots</u>

So many people are still using the non stick cookware with the toxic Teflon synthetic polymer without knowing about its dangers. Anything that is non stick in terms of cookware is not healthy to use and there are plenty of alternatives like stainless steel or cast iron. Yes using non stick cookware is more convenient, quicker and easier but at what price? Toxic fumes are released every time you heat up the pan even when the pan is in good condition and when it's old and scratched then you're just dousing yourself and your home in this chemical warfare agent known as PFIB, and a chemical analog of the WWII nerve gas phosgene. The health problems caused consist of heart disease, thyroid disease, Teflon flu from which many factory workers died and that resembles regular flu like symptoms with difficulty in breathing. Throw out all the non stick cookware and get replacements such as stainless steel or iron pans that cause no harm to you or your family.

<u>Plastics</u>

Plastic has made our lives easier in many and it's an affordable way to package and store things but the dangers of using plastic is now coming to the forefront and the realities aren't good. Although plastic is a cheaper alternative to glass or aluminum, the long term health risks don't make it worthwhile. When you look around your home you'll see plastic everywhere. All of your food is wrapped or packaged in plastic, you have plastic Tupperware, plastic trays and plates, medicine containers, plastic containers for all your shampoos and toiletries and plastic drinking bottles, plastic toys for your kids, plastic chairs and tables and so on. Obviously it's almost impossible to remove all plastic from your home but you can definitely minimize your exposure, especially when it comes to food container and items you touch often. Anything that sits in plastic for a long period of time that's edible should be first to go. Try purchasing products that are in glass containers whenever you can or alternatively have glass containers that you can transfer food to when you store them in the fridge. Plastic leaks carcinogen toxins that disrupt the hormones and poison the body and it gets more dangerous as the plastic ages or sits in a hot environment. Food products packaged in plastic are stored for long periods of time before they arrive to the store, often in hot conditions in warehouses and trucks although studies show that plastics leak toxins even when not in hot conditions so it's bad either way. All your plastic containers, Tupperware, plates, cooking utensils or cutlery should be thrown away. Any plastic drinking bottles (even the sport Nalgene ones that were once assumed safe) should not be used. There are now alternatives to everything in a non plastic material and aluminum drinking bottles are safe and just as lightweight.

Substances

Substances have been around for as long as time and almost everyone uses something at one time or another but it's mainly about finding a balance and choosing as natural a substance as possible so we can minimize the damage. Whether it's beer, cigarettes, marijuana or cocaine, using drugs of any kind on a regular basis isn't good for anyone. All substances wreck havoc on your nervous system, hormones and organ function. When a person uses substances to the point where they are dependent on them for relaxation, when they can't enjoy an activity without it or use it as a crutch before they can perform or socialize, it's an issue and must be addressed. Even if you're smoking one cigarette or drinking one drink a day, you might think that's not a lot but it adds up over long periods of time and still does damage. If you are using substances at large amounts for a long period of time then it will cause permanent damage to your body. If you are trying to reach ultimate health then you must cut out substances or at the very least take periodical breaks from it, use as natural a substance as possible (ie. organic alcohol or natural cigarettes) and then also try to lessen the intake.

The kitchen

No matter what you eat, in what shape, form or amount, one thing that everyone must do is remove as many toxins and chemicals from your food. Here I'm going to give you the dirty ten and if you can remove these items from your food even if you don't change one more thing about your diet or food intake, you will have already done your body so much wonders. Of course there are hundreds of toxic chemicals that you will find in food but these are the most widely used and the most harmful. If you decide to go fully organic 100% of the time then you'll be avoiding most of the unnatural chemicals but for now you should memorize this list and get familiar with these names. Make a list of these and place it on your fridge and keep a little list of them in your wallet so you can eliminate them one by one. Get used to checking the ingredient labels of produce when you shop. If you can avoid these then you will already be on your way to a healthier & happier you.

THE TOP TEN MOST DANGEROUS CHEMICALS:

1. SODIUM NITRATE

2. ARTIFICIAL SWEETENERS (ASPARTAME)

3. MONOSODIUM GLUTAMATE (MSG)

4. HIGH FRUCTOSE CORN SYRUP (HFCS)

5. HYDROGENATED OILS (TRANS FATS)

6. FOOD DYES/COLORS (YELLOW, RED, BLUE, GREEN..)

7. BHA & BHT & TBHQ

8. SULFUR DIOXIDE

9. POTASSIUM BROMATE

10. ARTIFICIAL FLAVOR

1. SODIUM NITRATE: *Found in hot dogs, bacon, cured meats, lunch meats, smoked fish, sausages, corned beef, processed meats.*

Sodium nitrate/nitrite is used to preserve meats and brighten their color as well as to make even old and lifeless meats look fresh and juicy. It's one of the most toxic ingredients you can find and once it enters your body it turns highly carcinogenic, enters the bloodstream and wreaks havoc with a number of internal organs: the liver and pancreas in particular. Sodium nitrite is widely regarded as a toxic ingredient, and was almost completely banned in the 1970's but was vetoed by food manufacturers and since has been flourishing on our plates.

2. ARTIFICIAL SWEETENERS: *Found in diet or sugar free sodas, jello, sugar free anything, baking goods, ice tea, toothpaste, pudding, cereal, breath mints and also as an alternative sweetener for sugar - NutraSweet, Equal.*

Found in almost everything that is diet, sugar free or low sugar, this artificial sweetener is a horrible carcinogenic that accounts for more adverse reactions than all other food combined. This lab made powder erodes intelligence, wrecks short-term memory and can lead to serious things like brain tumors, diabetes, lymphoma, multiple sclerosis, Alzheimer's, fibromyalgia, Parkinson's, migraines, seizures, depression, anxiety attacks and dizziness. Acesulfame-K which is newer than Aspartame should also be avoided.

3. MONOSODIUM GLUTAMATE: *Found in soups, salad dressings, sauces, chips, snacks, frozen dinners, Chinese food, cookies, seasonings and lunch meats.*

MSG is an amino acid used as a flavor enhancer or salt replacement in numerous items especially in restaurants. This additive is known as an excitotoxin, a substance which overexcites cells to the point of damage or death. Studies show that eating MSG can result in adverse side effects which include depression, disorientation, eye damage, fatigue, headaches and obesity. Consuming MSG also damages your neurological pathways of the brain especially the function that tells us when we're full which explains why people consuming MSG suffer from obesity.

4. HIGH FRUCTOSE CORN SYRUP: *Found in candy, bread, yogurt, sauces, salad dressing, canned vegetables and soup, cereal.*

This is a hard one to eliminate as it's pretty much found in everything, especially anything that's processed. High fructose corn syrup accounts for more calorie intake than any other item in America and this artificial sweetener causes tissue damage throughout the body, increases cholesterol and contributes to diabetes. It's also the fastest way to put on weight and it narrows the blood vessels which is very harmful for a variety of reason.

5. HYDROGENATED OIL: *Found in all fried foods, margarine, chips, crackers, cookies, baked goods, fast food.*

Although banned in many countries, here in the US this is widely used in so many food items. Hydrogenated anything is no good and when you see that word in the ingredient list you can be sure that it's a dangerous substance that does the body harm. Studies show that it increases cholesterol leading to heart attacks, increases inflammation throughout the body, causes strokes and heart disease and other major health problems.

6. FOOD DYES: *Found in candy, soft drinks, cereal, sports drinks, ice cream, fruit cocktail, macaroni and cheese, lemonade, salad dressing, American cheese.*

These artificial colorings that are seen in ingredients as food coloring, yellow#6, yellow tartrazine, Red#40, Blue#2

& Blue#1, contribute to a number of behavioral problems in children and leads to a reduction in IQ. Studies have shown that these artificial colorings are linked with cancer of all forms, cause permanent chromosomal damage, cause thyroid issues, brain-nerve transmission issues and kidney and adrenal tumors. Especially children as they are still in the development stages, must not consume anything with artificial coloring but you should avoid it too.

7. BHA, BHT & TBHQ: *Found in cereal, chewing gun, potato chips, vegetable oils, candy, frozen sausages, enriched rice, lard, jello, shortening.*

Butylated hydroxyanisole (BHA) and butylated hydrozyttoluene (BHT) are preservatives found in numerous food items. This common preservative keeps foods from losing it's color and going rancid. Regular consumption affects the neurological system of the brain, alters behavior and has potential to cause all forms of cancer. Tertiary Butylhydroquinone (TBHQ) is also a preservative which is a form of butane. Consuming as little as 1 gram of TBHQ can cause delirium, vomiting, nausea, collapse and ADHD and restlessness in children. Long term consumption has been linked with stomach cancers and estrogen imbalance in women.

8. SULFUR DIOXIDE: *Found in soft drinks, dried fruit, juices, cordials, wine, vinegar, beer, potato products.*

Also called E220, this toxic additive was banned from being used on raw vegetables and fruit by the FDA but is still widely available on other products. Consumption of this may result in bronchial problems, hypotension and destroys vitamin B1 and E and it's especially not recommended for consumption by children. The International Labour Organization says to avoid E220 if you suffer from conjunctivitis, bronchitis, emphysema, bronchial asthma, or cardiovascular disease.

9. POTASSIUM BROMATE: *Found in breads and baked goods.*

This chemical adds body to baked goods and breads and has been linked to all forms of cancers in animal studies. Eating even a small amount daily will have long term health risks.

10. ARTIFICIAL FLAVOR: *Found in all sorts of food items.*

This is a real evil one as it's a name that's used for over a 100 artificial additives that can hide behind this seemingly small and unimportant ingredient name. Eating tiny amounts of all sorts of cocktails of artificial chemicals that are made in a lab to taste like natural items will do major damage, cause allergic reactions and behavioral problems. One of them like Diacetyl which is used in butter on microwave popcorn has been linked with very dangerous lung disease called lymphocytic bronchiolitis that many factory workers died from. It's also known to be linked with Alzheimer's disease and neurological disturbance.

* * *

THE EXERCISE:

* Dispose of all the household cleaners you have in the home. Make home made cleaners or purchase natural, non toxic cleaners instead.

* Go through your medicine cabinet and dispose of anything you can make a commitment to never use again. Think about ailments you have often and do some research on natural remedies or home therapies. Then make sure you get whatever remedies you need ahead of time so you have those handy to try when sickness hits.

* Throw our your microwave, non stick cookware and any plastic containers, plastic water bottles or plastic items you can do away with that you have in the home.

* Go through all your toiletries and throw away everything unnatural. Replace them with home made or natural alternatives.

* If you take substances of any kind, write down your current commitment of either cutting it out or cutting down and be very specific. If you are not quitting completely then commit to consuming organic alcoholic beverages and natural cigarettes. Put this commitment up somewhere where you can see it every day.

* Go through your food in the kitchen and throw out anything containing any of the 10 toxic ingredients. Next time you go shopping visit a food store that has healthy options and as much organic products as possible and look for natural alternatives instead of the toxic food items you bought before.

* Make a list of the 10 dangerous additives and put this in your wallet. Make a commitment starting today that you will memorize these one by one and check the ingredients when shopping. Do not consume chemicals as this is directly poisoning you. If you CAN commit to go organic then know that this would be best and then you would not have to worry yourself with checking labels as much.

STEP TWO

Detox the body

When you have a toxic body that is filled with a large amount of backed up poisons, you cannot function at your best and disease is imminent. Eventually you realize this and are ready to change your eating and lifestyle habits but unfortunately at that toxic level it's not enough to just make some changes and a detox is necessary before the change of lifestyle is implemented. For most people, by the time they realize that they should eat better and take better care of themselves, they've done enough damage and put their bodies through so much abuse that they have to take stronger measures to clean things up. The body, as resilient as it is, if it's been fed toxins for many years causing a massive back up of all systems, will need a huge kick start so it can begin flushing the junk and garbage out. You want to get your body as close to the perfect state as you can and you want to get it to a point where you can start fresh. It's just like cleaning a really messy house that's getting a make over that's stacked with trash from ceiling to floor. The first step is to remove all the trash, strip the place of whatever doesn't serve it and that's when you will actually have space to work and rebuild. When you have an empty and clean house then you can give it a fresh coat of paint, give it some touch ups and start adding in all the materials you do like and bringing in furniture that looks great. If you don't remove any of the trash from the run down house and aren't willing to clean it but still bring in all the nice furniture and set it up all between the trash inside then you won't notice much of the change. This is why the steps you take must be in order and before you start eating healthy, you must get rid off the junk that's been clogging your body up for years. No matter how you choose to detox, you must flush out all the built up toxins before you begin refueling and rebuilding. Depending on your history and how bad your health is, you might be great with only one cleanse, but if you're in really bad shape and you've abused your body for a long period of time then you should set up a few cleanses for yourself, completing one every month for three months or so.

There are numerous ways to cleanse and I'm sure you might have heard of some of them from celebrities, friends and magazines. The list is endless with everything from the cabbage soup diet, the master cleanse, paleo diet, eating raw, gluten free and of course hundreds of pills, powders, shakes and meal replacements. A person can become overwhelmed and confused while trying each one here and there and trying to figure out which one is fact or fiction can be tiring as most are just a fad or fashion. I hear about a new diet or pill regularly and although of course new health products will always arrive on the market, I prefer to stick to something that has been around for a long time and is 100% natural. I will share my favorite ways to detox but no matter what cleanse you choose to do, the main thing is to be committed to the process. Doing a cleanse without following through isn't going to give you the results you are looking for and doing a cleanse for a day or two will not put a dent in the major overhaul that your body needs. The detox is the least fun part of these steps so if you start then make sure you finish otherwise you're just wasting time and effort. You must be serious, take this step with dedication and commit. Once you are actually detoxing, know that the process will not feel good as all the horrible things you've eaten and put into your body your entire life will suddenly be coming out of you in a matter of days. How can you not expect to feel ill from that? Don't let this frighten or worry you as this is expected and normal. That's how you know that the detox process is working. The more toxic you are, the worse you will feel during the cleanse so take refuge in knowing that you are seeing results if you're detoxing and you are feeling all the symptoms of toxins leaving your body. Remember that once you go through it, you'll be a healthier person in the end. People often give up only a third of the way in because the symptoms get too severe or because they get scared as they feel so horrible that they convince themselves that this surely cannot be good for them. So before you start, understand the process and really commit to the detox and expect to feel uncomfortable symptoms. This is hands down the most misunderstood fact about cleansing so please take note that you are NOT supposed to feel good during a cleanse. Detoxing is a process in which there are built up toxins that are breaking down and leaving your body and this is difficult and will have symptoms that will leave you feeling sickly, ill, in pain, nauseous and so on so expect this. To cleanse you also have to give up a lot of your normal routine, so no more dinners with friends and all the other social events that include food and drink. You have to plan ahead and prepare for all the situations that you will have to avoid and put off. You can do anything you put your mind to so no matter how difficult it is, push through, maybe put together a support system of friends or family who can give you inspiration when you want to give up. Know that anytime your mind is telling you to stop it's just your fears talking as well as the addiction to sugars. When the chemicals and poisons are leaving your body you will not feel great but afterwards you will feel like a new person. Be patient and go through the process and know that you can have the will power if you really want it.

HOW TO DETOX:

There are many ways to detox or cleanse a body but I've listed the few ways I recommend doing it. Detoxing naturally without adding more toxins to the body is very important so you must avoid any cleanses where taking teas, pills or powders is part of it. It's also important to use organic and fresh foods and juices at that time. I believe that any cleanses that require you to put pills, vitamins, powders or teas into your body are a backward way of cleansing as even the most healthy natural herb can be seen as a toxin that clogs up your body at this sensitive time.

WATER FASTING:

The best and most efficient way to detox is to water fast although this takes a lot of will power and mental strength. Water fasting has been practiced for thousands of years and although there are western doctors and specialists who like to denounce it as a dangerous process, it's one of the most natural and safest processes that exist in nature. If you wish to read more in depth about water fasting then you can most definitely do some researching and reading as there are so many books on the history and birth of it but I will spare my readers from going into lengthy explanations of how or where it originated. Animals in the wild will instinctively water fast when sick completely abstaining from food. Young children do it naturally too if they don't feel well but of course that's until we force feed them chicken soup and pills and syrups and even adults will naturally have no appetite when ill. Our bodies are incredibly smart and they know it's not good to be processing food when trying to heal, fight off a disease or regenerate. Abstaining from food for long enough will eventually shut down your digestive system which takes about 2 to 3 days, after which the body will natural enter the actual 'fasting' period. The body is programmed to use the least important parts of itself for energy so it starts using up areas of the body as fuel, beginning with the stored fat reserves as well as eventually using other unnecessary masses and tumors. People have fasted not just for days but for weeks and months at a time and it shouldn't be feared but obviously proper techniques and precautions should be followed. Disease can truly be eradicated if water fasting is executed correctly over periods of time and the only real danger is if you reach the starvation phase when the body has used up all the unnecessary masses and begins using the vital organs as food but this would never happen during a 7 or 10 day fast and would pertain to a very lengthened fast when the body mass index falls drastically, hence why supervision is recommended for long fasts. When water fasting is used to combat a very serious illness then supervision is also recommended as those fasts can last many months. An incredible amount of people with incurable cancers and illnesses have been cured through water fasting and although that's a long process, doing a short water fast purely for cleansing purposes is safe and easy to do at home. The medical community and pharmaceutical industry have spent lots of money and effort in keeping water fasting and it's magical effects secret as it would greatly damage their reputation and income should this be revealed to the masses but if you really want to find out about what miracles it's done for thousands of people around the world then you will find plenty of documentation on it. If you are worried about doing your first water fast on your own then you can contact a holistic practitioner who can assist you or guide you via phone should you wish to have someone experienced answer any questions or issues that come up. In my opinion, water fasting is one of the most magical ways you can heal and detox your body and although there are many other ways to cleanse, this is definitely the fastest and deepest way. Although water fasting is incredibly safe, as I mentioned before, there are still proper steps to be followed that will help and enhance the process. If you are generally healthy, not pregnant and are doing a 7 to 10 day fast then you can most definitely do this at home.

To do a water fast at home you will need a minimum of seven days. Doing a fast for a shorter period isn't worthwhile and not recommended as it takes your body two to three days to get to the actual 'fasting' stage. I would personally recommend anything between 7 and 10 days at home for your first water fast. Although some have water fasted while still working, I highly advise against this and believe that taking time off work and being in a peaceful environment is really important during a fast, otherwise you will only reap a small amount of the benefits. If you cannot take off work and plan to be running about then you should look into another means of cleansing as water fasting makes a person slightly weak, dizzy and light headed. When you are fasting your body should be resting at all times so if you are doing too much activity then the body is using the energy for that activity instead of the healing it should be doing. During the water fast it's important to begin it correctly and to break the fast correctly. Entering the fast or beginning it isn't as strict and you can honestly begin a fast at any second but breaking it incorrectly can land you in trouble especially if you do something silly like have a huge steak dinner right after you're done fasting. Remember that re-starting your digestive system must be done with caution and eating small amounts of only raw vegetables and fruits is the only way you can break it. If you eat any meat or processed food immediately after your fast then it can clog your stomach and truly give you one of the worst tummy aches or even send you to the hospital so take care to follow the directions after your fast. Below I've written out very clear and basic instructions for your home water fast.

First you must decide when you will be fasting ahead of time and commit to that date. Make sure you don't have any trips, birthdays, weddings or other important events around that time and take the time off work. If you use your vacation days it will be the best way you've spent them so don't feel guilty for taking the time off for you and your body. After settling on a date, begin preparing with the elimination of food a week before the fast as doing this will insure your fast will be much easier with less withdrawal symptoms and headaches. Doing this is optional and if you feel that a week is not something you can commit to doing as preparation then do three days which will be good enough. Remember that the more days you can prepare, the easier your fast will be. The more food you can eliminate, the less symptoms you will have as often the headaches you feel during fasting is caused by the withdrawal of caffeine, sugar and other food items.

Preparing for a water fast at home:

Three to seven days before your scheduled fast is to begin, start preparing by cutting the following from your diet;

* meat & animal products

* eggs

* all dairy (cheese, yogurt, butter, cream...)

* caffeine

* alcohol

* sugar

* junk food and processed food

Really do your best to remove as much of the list above as possible and try to eat a really healthy diet as this will help your body to transition to just water without too much shock. If you are drinking coffee, eating sugars and junk food the day before your water fast then you are going to suffer a lot more than you need to as the withdrawal from all of those will be severe. Try your best to stick to a vegetarian, fresh and healthy diet before the fast to flush the body and intestines as much as you can. This is the time to prepare your body and mind for the fast. Another great idea is to make the portions smaller and smaller as you get closer to the fast so you're not stuffing yourself right before your water fast.

Example of things to eat during the preparation:

Breakfast: granola, fruit.

Snack: nuts & smoothie.

Lunch: salad, raw veggies dipped in hummus, soup.

Dinner: steamed vegetables (change up the variety every evening to include different nutrients), baked sweet potato.

Snack: herbal tea & dried fruit.

During the preparation you should also wean yourself off any medications or pills you might currently be taking as you cannot be taking medications when water fasting. If you are on medications that are vital which you cannot stop taking then a water fast isn't right for you. You should consult your doctor or specialist before stopping medications if you are not sure. Fasting while pregnant is also not allowed.

The day before your begin your water fast I would recommend making numerous veggie juices. If you don't have a juicer at home then try to find a local juice shop but ONLY drink juices made from organic vegetables. The day before the fast you should try to consume as little solid food as possible so that the transition into the fast is smoother. Soups, stews and broths are great but a light salad won't hurt either. Please avoid meat or other complex food items for dinner the night before as your last few meals will sit in your intestines since your bowl movements will stop once you begin the fast. The day before your fast is the most important so this is the time you need to avoid all the things I listed before.

Choosing a good place to water fast is also very important so avoid an environment that is stressful or loud. Being in a place that makes you feel safe, that is peaceful and calm is essential. If you live with other people then take the time to explain to them about what you will be doing so you have their understanding and support. Don't be put off doing a water fast if your family or friends don't understand the process and don't be scared by comments such as 'you will die if you don't eat for seven days!', this is just ignorance speaking. For obvious reasons you cannot be around anyone who will be cooking food as the smell will drive you nuts! If you live alone then clean out your fridge and pack up any food items you can if you think you will be tempted to eat something. Ask people living with you to avoid cooking during that time and also discuss with them your needs regarding having a quiet place to water fast. Make sure you prepare well and have everything you will need during that time, such as filtered water, to last the length of the fast. If you don't have a great living situation that is stress free or peaceful then look into going away somewhere tranquil to do your water fast or alternatively find a water fasting clinic. Often getting away from your home environment will make it easier to complete the fast.

Before you begin your water fast, you must make sure that you have an unlimited amount of clean water. I discuss what good quality water means in the next chapter so refer to that and whatever you do, DO NOT drink water from plastic or from the tap while fasting. Your body is extremely sensitive during a water fast and drinking really clean water is crucial. Chemicals will leak from the plastic bottles into the water and tap water has a lot of added chemicals as well so neither one of those is a great choice. It's important to find the healthiest and cleanest filtered or spring water for your water fast as this will be the only thing you'll be putting into your body for the entire length of the fast. Make sure you are drinking plenty water throughout the day while fasting and don't chug huge amounts of water once a day but drink every 20 minutes or as you're thirsty. There isn't a perfect pre-set amount of water you should be drinking so listen to your body but take note of how many glasses you're drinking and if it's less than six a day then that might be too little. Somewhere between 6 and 10 glasses is great but I urge you to listen to your body as different climate, different body mass and many other variables make it impossible to set an amount that everyone can follow.

While water fasting you will get light headed and dizzy so be very careful when walking around and take a few breaths in and out and hold onto something when standing up from a sitting or laying position as a lot of people water fasting will faint when standing too quickly.

Also make sure you don't spend all day long staring at the computer as this is tiring on your eyes and brain. Checking your email once in a while or watching a movie is okay but remember that the body working it's hardest at flushing toxins out when you are truly resting. Reading is a good way to pass the time as well as anything that doesn't require too much energy. Exercise of any kind is discouraged as you don't want to expel energy onto something other than healing. Light walks and gentle stretching are alright. I also highly recommend 15 to 20 minutes of sunlight exposure every day when you are fasting as the sun has great healing properties and a source of much needed vitamin D. Make sure you do not wear sunscreen as that defeats the purpose of the sun exposure and lay out in either early morning or late afternoon when the sun will not be too hot or intolerable. Wear as little clothing as possible while sunbathing so that you can have sunlight exposure to as much of your body as possible and don't stay in the sun for longer than 30 minutes. Again, be careful when standing up after laying in the sun as the light and heat can make you even more dizzy.

Initially the first two days you will feel very hungry but the hunger will diminish by the third day when the actual fasting process begins. You will notice that your hunger will subside completely by the end of the third day as you enter the true fasting phase and this is when you will start feeling the detox begin to work as you'll start seeing the symptoms of the toxins leaving your body. Everyone experiences different symptoms depending on how toxic you are and depending on what food you have been consuming recently. If you feel incredibly harsh symptoms then try to take comfort in knowing that the detox is working and that you have a lot of elimination to go through. This isn't a reason to be panicked, it's simply a sign that everything is going as it should. Some people experience very mild symptoms with only a few headaches and others harsher ones with extreme lower back pain and vomiting. Mostly the symptoms include a combination of headaches and nausea, but other side effects can include vomiting, diarrhea, constipation, body aches, back pain, trembling, break outs or rashes, developing flu or cold symptoms, insomnia and fever chills. It will generally feel as if you are detoxing or going through a withdrawal of a drug and that's because many of the toxins and chemicals that leave the body at this time are exactly that. The period of fasting becomes a waiting game where you have to accept that you must go through whatever side effects you experience coming up but that eventually they will pass. There is no short cut or easy way to eliminate this junk from your body and most of it has spent months, years or a lifetime being stored. Certain symptoms pass as certain toxins leave your body and then new symptoms might pop up. During a water fast you should expect your breath to smell horrible, to have an unpleasant body odor and to pass odd stools that might be of alarming color or smell. If you can have a water fasting expert on call via email or phone, it's a great way to put your mind at ease in case you have questions or concerns. Often this isn't costly and gives you the peace of mind that everything is going according to plan.

No matter how bad your breadth or body odor smells, remember that it is the toxins leaving your body and you must avoid putting any chemicals on at this time so do not use any toiletries whatsoever unless you absolutely have to use a small amount of all natural soap and even this in moderation. DO NOT use fragrances, deodorants perfumes, toothpaste (as tiny amounts will be swallowed when you brush your teeth and will re-start your digestive system which will stop the fasting process), creams, mouthwash, lotions or make up. I recommend taking daily warm showers or baths and scrubbing your skin with a natural loofah as that accelerates the detox process and helps eliminate toxins via the skin. Our skin is the largest organ and it's a great tool for elimination so doing daily body scrubs are incredible for you during a fast.

Another important factor that many forget is to really not consume anything or put anything, no matter how small, in your mouth during the fast. If you start chewing a mint or gum, you will immediately halt the fasting process. Even something as simple as chewing on a plain toothpick is not allowed. The moment you begin chewing, even if you are not swallowing anything, the digestion process is booted up in your stomach as the digestion process begins in the mouth when we begin the action of chewing. This action will stop the fasting immediately. If you do eat anything, you will suddenly feel your hunger and appetite returning and you will have to water fast again from the beginning, again having to wait another 2 or 3 days to reach the fasting phase. So remember that nothing goes in your mouth at all, including toothpaste. Brush your teeth with a toothbrush and water and avoid anything else. If you do end up eating anything accidentally then you must re-start your water fasting from day one again .

As the days of your water fast pass by, you'll notice that it gets easier and for most part the worst side effect is boredom. We are so used to being super busy that it becomes almost painful to sit around doing nothing but keep reminding yourself that you are resting and healing your body. It's your job to relax and allow your body to work it's magic. Eventually, no matter how long and tedious it might seem, the days will pass and you will come to the end of your week or ten day water fast. During your fast it can be a great time to meditate, reflect upon your life, catch up on lots of sleep and reading. You can have friends come by and keep you company or catch up with relatives who live far away via the phone. Give this time to your body and your mind and turn off the world so you can experience no stress and no distractions.

As much as it's important to prepare before the fast, breaking your fast correctly is even more vital. You can do quite a bit of damage by eating too quickly or eating the incorrect diet after your water fast which can cause severe stomach pain and discomfort so take care to break the fast very slowly and carefully. Once you begin eating you are re-starting your digestive system so don't shock it by having a huge meal. After a water fast you should only consume absolute natural items that are plucked straight from the earth and close to the source, such as fruit and vegetables. I suggest breaking the fast with a few pieces of watermelon as it's the easiest to digest and consists mainly of water. Eat a small piece of watermelon and make sure to chew it very well and then eat a few more pieces every hour. You will notice that your hunger will suddenly return and you might have a huge appetite but avoid going into a frenzy of eating and stick to the plan. After eating water melon for the first half of the day, you can then introduce some other fruits of your choosing for the second half, just make sure they are ripe and organic. Do not stuff yourself and make sure you chew everything really well. That evening after eating watermelon and other fruits throughout the day, you can make a veggie broth. To make a veggie broth chop up a bunch of organic and fresh vegetables, as little as two or as many as you like. Please avoid frozen, canned or pre-cooked vegetables, use only fresh ones! After you chop them up into small pieces, boil them in a pot of filtered water until they are all very tender. Don't add any spices, sauces or salt and just enjoy the vegetable broth on it's own just as is.

On the second day you can start eating all fruit and vegetables whenever you feel hungry. Drinking freshly made veggie juices is also great as you're pumping a concentrate of nutrients into your body. Take your time and really enjoy raw vegetables especially, make a little salad with lettuce, grated carrots, bell peppers and any other veggies you like with squeezed lemon juice over it. Suddenly you'll be able to taste vegetables in a whole new light as water fasting will have cleansed your taste buds and opened you up to a whole new world.

Ultimately, the first two days you want to stick to only fresh fruits and vegetables and nothing else. Eating meat, bread, dairy or processed foods at this time will not only hurt your tummy but it will immediately clog up your body which is such a waste after having done such a wonderful cleaning. This is when your body is most sensitive and everything is flowing and open. Your body needs you to feed it natural and quality nutrients at this time. There will be a massive hunger surge when you begin eating but make sure you don't overeat, as this will stretch out your stomach so stick to many small meals throughout the day. By the third day you can slowly introduce your regular diet but I would recommend that you try to be as healthy as possible for as long as you can immediately after the water fast as this is when you can really rebuild you body. Every cell and organism is now screaming for nutrition so do your best and you can literally renew everything at this time.

JUICING:

The second way to detox and probably the most popular way is to do a juicing cleanse. This is somewhat easier than a water fast and allows you to still function in your day to day life so you can keep working, keep driving and do your daily chores. A lot of people cannot take time off work to water fast so this is a great alternative way to detox without having to put everything on hold. During a juice cleanse I still recommend as much rest as you can possibly get and in my juicing programs I offer in Los Angeles I insist that everyone rests most of the time. When juicing you pump large quantities of really fresh nutrients into your body which would be impossible to match if you ate the vegetables. When a vegetable is juiced you remove the fiber ultimately being able to fit five servings of vegetables in just one juice! Juicing also cuts you off from the solid food intake, giving your digestive system a much needed rest. The combination of those two actions create a great detox system that allows for poisons to break down and be eliminated from the body. There are numerous juicing programs popping up all over the country but be careful of buying expensive juicing programs where you're drinking juices that weren't freshly made. A juice made yesterday will not have the same benefits as a freshly made juice because the enzymes and nutrients die as the time passes. Also beware of juicing companies that cut their juices with water to save money, MOST juicing detox companies that sell packaged juice cleanses cut their juices with water so why pay money for something that's not fresh and not 100% juice?

When you are juicing on your own at home it's pretty simple and I believe there aren't too many rules to follow except for a few so if you follow those then it's pretty simple and easy as long as you have the will power.

The biggest mistake that I see people make with juicing is that they allow fruit to be too prominent in each serving. Fruit has it's benefits but that's when you are consuming it as a whole so when you juice a fruit and remove the fiber, you are left with mostly sugar. Yes it is natural sugar, in it's natural state, but sugar nonetheless. When people are doing a juicing program and drinking four juices a day, pumping that much sugar into your body in liquid form can really add up to an amount that does the body harm. Of course some vegetable juices are hardly drinkable without a lemon or grapefruit but the more you can stick to vegetables the better. I would never recommend putting a whole lemon or one whole apple in one serving of juice, instead try a quarter or a half in a serving. Your ratio should be 90% vegetables and 10% fruit and definitely NEVER less than 80% vegetables per juice.

Another mistake I see people make is that they get stuck on the same two vegetables of their choice and they juice the same thing over and over. Although all vegetables are good for you, remember that each vegetable has a different set of nutrients, a different purpose and a different effect. When you juice only those same few vegetables throughout the week, you get those nutrients but you are missing out on a world of others. A great way to make sure you include all varieties is to have a list of all the vegetables that are available in your area and you want to make sure you go through the list and juice as many as you can during your cleanse. The more vegetables you include, the better and there are hardly any vegetables that you cannot juice! Make sure you don't stray away from vegetables that you don't know or don't like. In fact you should specifically juice the vegetables you don't know or like as those probably contain the vitamins your body has been missing. You can read so much information about a certain vegetable and what it does for your body if you need inspiration. For example, you probably never eat dandelions but buy a bunch and juice them to specifically create a deep detox of the liver.

When you are making your own juices at home, remember that you will have to use one vegetable that makes a lot of juice as a base. Celery, cucumbers, carrots are great examples of vegetables you can use as a base as they make a decent amount of juice whereas something like spinach will give you a few tablespoons of juice from a large bunch. The base vegetable will make up around 50% of your juice and then you top it off with a few other vegetables to make the other half. Again you shouldn't always use the same vegetable for a base but keep changing it up. A lot of people ask about what vegetables you should choose to juice and honestly you can juice any vegetables as long as you include a variety. I especially recommend juicing vegetables that you maybe never eat so that you can fill up on the nutrients you might be missing. A great detox is also thinking about doing a green juice only the entire time so that means sticking to mainly green vegetables as those have the most detoxifying qualities.

I would recommend drinking four 16 ounce juices per day with water in between to avoid dehydration. Make sure you don't drink all your juices in the morning or all at night but spread them out evenly throughout the day. Unless you're using a cold press juicer, drink the juices that you made that day and don't pre-make the juices for the next day as the nutrient content decreases over time. If you're very busy and don't have the time to make them fresh as you go then make your juices in the morning and refrigerate them. The juices will last and be alright to drink through the day if stored in a fridge, but if you're at home and can make the juices fresh then do that as it intensifies the benefits. ALWAYS use organic produce when juicing as juicing a non organic vegetable only makes a cocktail of the pesticides that were on the vegetable adding to your toxicity. Juicing a non organic vegetable should never be a compromise. If you get your juices at a local juice shop make sure they make them fresh and that they use organic produce. Buying pre-made juices in plastic bottles does not justify a juice cleanse! V8 and other bottled juices DO NOT count as a fresh vegetable juices! Anything that comes pasteurized and packaged in a bottle that lasts for a week or longer is not a good tool for detoxing during a juicing program.

If you have the money and the time then I would recommend doing a juice program at a retreat as it's easier when the the juices are made for you. It also helps when you are surrounded by others going through the same program and as well as being in a relaxing environment away from home, work, friends and distractions. Often completing any sort of detox program at home on your own can be challenging and that's why a lot of people invest in going away to do this. Although if you're dedicated then it is very possible on your own.

Just like with water fasting, you must commit to a date ahead of time and mark it down in your calendar. Look forward to it instead of dreading it like a jail sentence, it's for your health after all! Before you start make sure you commit to the amount of days you will juice for and don't change this during the program. Remember that a minimum of 5 days is recommended but you can juice as long as two weeks. I also recommend avoiding heavy exercise regiments, I recommend being in a relaxing environment, resting as much as possible, sunlight exposure daily and not taking part in stressful work and other activities.

DIET CLEANSE:

If both water fasting and juicing scares you beyond belief and going without solid food isn't an option then you can do a cleanse while still eating food. I must stress that this is the mildest form of cleansing and isn't nearly as good or as proactive but for some this is the only option so it's still better than nothing. If you are very ill or severely toxic then I must highly recommend that you complete a water fast or juice cleanse as this might not be as efficient in removing large quantities of built up junk. Doing a cleanse using food is probably the most difficult also as you'll be tempted to push the boundaries of what's allowed that's why it's very important to be very clear on the rules. Keep in mind that if you cheat, you are only cheating yourself. Remember that doing any program without being committed not only wastes your time but also forces you to go through the work without reaping the benefits so make sure you are ready and do whatever you need to feel inspired whether it's using post it notes, support from a friend or vision boards of your goals.

The simple rules of a diet cleanse is that you will consume nothing else but RAW vegetables and a small amount of fruit. If during the cleanse you consume mainly fruits and hardly any vegetables then you will not cleanse your body at all. Your diet should consist of 10% fruit and the rest all vegetables. Now you might ask 'how can I only eat vegetables? But then just remind yourself that the alternative is drinking veggie juices or water fasting and be happy to munch on that platter of baby carrots, cabbage and bell peppers.

I want to answer the frequently asked questions I receive about what is considered a vegetable or allowed in the diet cleanse. The following food items are NOT vegetables and should not be consumed during this cleanse - nuts, seeds, beans, lentils, olive oil, salt, pepper, salad dressing, tea, rice, spices or cereal. I know you might want to argue about some of these and I've even had someone try to explain that pizza is mostly vegetables but to do this you must stick to the plan which is ONLY vegetables and ONLY raw vegetables and very little fruit. There might be lots of other healthy food items but that's not what this cleanse is about. It's about only putting LIVE foods into your body that are in their natural state.

During the diet cleanse, eating a variety of vegetables is important so don't avoid any vegetables and don't stick to eating the same two. You know that weird root thing you've seen at the store but have no idea what it is? This is the time to try it! You will get bored of eating raw vegetables and you will feel incredible withdrawals from sugar, caffeine, carbohydrates, alcohol and other junk foods but that's supposed to happen. Prepare yourself mentally before hand and expect that the cleanse is the hardest step. If you need to cut the vegetables into cute happy shapes that's okay, if you need to grate them or make them into a smoothie or just munch on the vegetables as they are, all that matters is that you get them down and don't starve yourself. Please don't go all week just eating one vegetable either but eat a variety to get as much and as many different types of nutrients.

To do a diet cleanse you must commit to a minimum of five days but I would recommend doing a week or ten days. Do as much as you possibly can as every day will do wonders for you. Many people have asked about cooking the vegetables and some surely do have difficulties digesting raw vegetables but you probably already know that cooking kills the nutrients especially when frying or boiling at high heat. Since frying is out as you cannot use oil or butter and boiling truly kills every live aspect of the vegetable, if you absolutely MUST cook some vegetables, I suggest that you only do so for one of your meals in the day. So eat raw vegetables and fruits for breakfast and lunch and throughout the day for snacking and then for dinner STEAM your vegetables. Steaming involves cooking with the least amount of damage to the vegetable leaving most of the nutrients still intact. Make sure you don't over steam the vegetables, leaving them to have a little crunch to them and also only steam one meal a day. Frying, boiling or baking is out of the question.

Besides these three methods I've outlined above I don't recommend any other forms of detoxing. There are lots of powders and shakes and teas and pills that promise to cleanse your body and although some of them are beneficial in some ways, as a whole, I prefer to use natural means to cleanse. This in my opinion is the absolute best way to clean your body and adding powders, teas or herbs to your body just adds to your toxicity levels as you don't know the quality of these powders, how they were produced, how long they were stored before they reached you, what chemicals were used, how the herb was extracted and so forth. When you buy a fresh organic produce you can see exactly what it is so I believe adding a powder to your water or drinking a pill every day can never ever replace a real natural live food.

*   *   *

THE EXERCISE:

Spend a good amount of time thinking about which detox plan is best for you and which one you can commit to. Once you choose the best plan for you, set up a date of when you will begin the cleanse and how many days you will cleanse for. Unless you have a set in stone very special event coming up, you should commit to setting up your detox to begin within two weeks of today. The best would be as soon as possible so avoid making excuses or procrastinating and just do it. Do not push this exercise off for the next three months as there should be nothing more important that your health. If you cannot take off work to do a water fast now and can only do that in six months then commit to doing a juice cleanse now or in the upcoming few weeks.

Write down all the details and make a list of everything you will need for your cleanse. Make sure you purchase everything you need ahead of time so you don't stress yourself out on the morning you're meant to begin your detox by not having things you need. Set up a support system during this time if you have close friends or family living near you. You must commit at this time and don't keep pushing the date later because of work meetings, dinners, birthdays or other "special" events. You doing a cleanse for your health and your body IS special.

* UNTIL YOU HAVE COMPLETED A CLEANSE OF YOUR CHOICE, DO NOT MOVE ONTO THE NEXT CHAPTER.

STEP THREE

Fuel your body correctly

After eliminating poisons from your home and doing a cleanse, you are now ready for the next step towards a healthier you. This is the part that will start rebuilding every cell, tissue and organ in your body and will reverse damage and reverse aging. Most of us have been consuming such low quality foods for so many years that every single one of us is deficient in multiple nutrients. After cleansing, your body is open and ready to receive the nutrition it really yearns for, so give it the right fuel it needs and it will reward you with true health, energy, a clear mind and balanced hormones. Fueling your body correctly will lead to the break down of disease and prevention of disease. You will live longer, you will enjoy a quality life and you will have less emotional, physical and mental issues.

WATER:

We will start with the most important factor - WATER. Many of you will be tempted to skip this chapter as you are tired of hearing and reading about water but I really hope you don't as water is vital to being healthy. The reason it's so important is that without correctly hydrating your body there is no way anything can function at an optimal and healthy level. Being chronically dehydrated all the time puts all your organs and body functions under immense strain. If you want your body to function well, be able to assimilate nutrients that you eat and constantly flush out toxins that you ingest, then you need to make water your best friend. You need to have water next to you when you sleep, take water with you everywhere you go and have it on hand at all times. Accept that 70% of your body is water and if the 70% isn't healthy and balanced then there is no way that the other 30% will make up for that.

Unless you live in one of the few places in the world where your tap water is known for being incredibly clean, you need to stop drinking tap water for good. Tap water has so many unnatural chemicals that don't belong in water that it's no wonder all of us are sick and with the federal laws that regulate tap water being so out of date, there isn't much hope for a change. Almost all tap water has fluoride added which is harmful to your health and it contains tiny amounts of hundreds of chemicals and contaminants that damage your body and make it impossible to stay healthy. Tap water is always acidic and drinking acidic water combined with eating an acidic diet, which most of us consume, makes for a highly acidic body in which disease thrives in. Metals are also commonly found in tap water which accumulate in your organs and do so much harm. The EPA and Congress regulate over 100 pollutants and 91 chemicals through the Safe Drinking Water Act but they admit that the water pollution law enforcement is unacceptably low. Most chemicals and toxins are legally allowed to be dumped into tap water as long as they stay under certain amounts so we are not only drinking water with fluoride and metals but we are also drinking a large cocktail of chemicals and contaminants. I highly recommend that you never drink tap water again. Also it's a myth that boiling your tap water removes the chemicals and makes it safe to drink. Boiling does not remove chemicals, it only removes bacteria so you should be using clean water to also make your tea, coffee, soups and so on. Don't use tap water for anything and if you have the money then I recommend getting a water filtration system for your entire home.

When people realize that tap water isn't good for them then they choose another alternative which they think is safer or healthier and that is buying water in plastic bottles or containers. Some even buy many cases of plastic water bottles and don't consume any other water besides that. This isn't a good choice at all due to plastic being highly toxic especially the plastic that is used in water bottles. The plastic leaks chemicals into the drinking water and it's detrimental to the environment. The water sold in plastic bottles has often been bottled long ago and most sit in overheated warehouses for long periods of time and then sit in overheated delivery trucks. Plastic is already highly toxic and plastic water bottles that have been exposed to really hot temperatures for weeks or possibly months while being stored just multiply in their toxicity levels. Never should there be an excuse to consume any liquid from plastic bottles and you should only purchase water from glass containers or bottles. You might think that avoiding plastic water bottles is impossible but it really isn't that difficult especially with some planning and forethought. If you are working this hard to get healthy then make a commitment to never drink from plastic again. Once you make the change to drinking healthier water, you will never look back and you will feel the difference.

Lately there has also been a trend to drink reverse osmosis water or alkaline water and this is nothing but a trend that's anything but natural. Reserve osmosis is a technique that strips the water of all the chemicals and additives but it also strips the water of all the natural elements and minerals which are essential to us. Reserve osmosis puts the water through a machine and process that truly kills the water so instead of it being a live mineral water, it becomes a stale dead liquid that we keep pumping into our system with no health benefits whatsoever. Reverse osmosis water also causes a build up of metals in the body as it's filtered through metal plates that leak metals into the water during the filtration process. This process changes the actual make up of water and our bodies no longer recognize it as water, forcing us to drink more than we actually need yet never truly hydrating our bodies as it's dead water instead of live water. Alkaline water is even worse as there is no machine that makes the water alkaline naturally. These machines add chemicals and powders to the water to make it alkaline changing the way the water particles behave, completely confusing the body. If you're drinking alkaline water made by a machine then you are just putting more toxins into the body. Unless you are drinking water that is naturally alkaline, from a spring in the ground then it's no good as it's unnatural.

You might be wondering what water you should be drinking and what water is healthy water. Well there are two options that you are left with and that's either to drink natural spring water or to buy a good water filter. Finding natural spring water isn't difficult no matter where you reside as companies exist all over the country that deliver large jugs to your home each month for a much cheaper price than buying small plastic water bottles. This might be pricier than tap water of course but since your body is 70% water and you want to find lasting health then that water should be as clean and as good as you can get it. Skipping this part and drinking toxic water is nothing but a slow form of poisoning oneself. Natural spring water comes out of the ground and it's alive, refreshing, healthy, naturally pH balanced and has all the minerals that we require in it. You wonder why people are deficient in minerals as we're meant to get a good amount of those in our water but tap, distilled and reverser osmosis water do not contain any minerals, only added metals and chemicals. If you're eating healthy, exercising, spending time in nature, breathing good air, meditating and doing everything right but you're drinking bad water then you are still doing 70% of it wrong and you will invite disease into your life. I recommend everyone start with putting great quality water into your body and invest in your health as drinking healthy and clean water is very important. It might be more money than you are willing to spend but if you can't invest in water then you will not have the absolute basic foundation of good health. A lot of spring water is sold in small glass bottles (make sure to buy glass when you can) but of course that's even more expensive so try to find a great spring water company that ships, delivers or sells larger bottles of spring water in gallons. I buy Mountain Valley Spring water and have it delivered to my home every month which is really convenient. You can also research if there are natural springs near you that sell cheaper water. The other option of getting a quality filtration system for your home is a great investment if you can afford it and if not then look into smaller water filters that you can use for drinking water. A lot of the very cheap water filters don't really get everything out of the water so invest in one that's rated well and lasts a lifetime. Do your research and buy the best water filter system you can afford.

The next thing after you've figured out your healthy water, is to buy one or two small water bottles (aluminum or glass) that you can take with you whenever you leave the house. Whether going to work or on errands, get in the habit of always filling up your bottle and taking it with you. Even if you're going out only for a few hours, bring your water. To avoid dehydration one must drink water every 20 minutes and although this might seem much at first, the more you can hydrate, the better. Don't make the mistake of not drinking water for six hours and then drinking large amounts afterwards as this will not prevent dehydration. Drinking throughout the day and constantly is important.

Once you change to healthy spring water or filtered water, you will notice that you will not need to drink as much to feel hydrated and you should also notice improvements in your energy levels, as well as the quality of your skin, hair and everything else.

ORGANIC:

A Lithuanian holistic health practitioner Ann Wigmore once said 'food can be either the safest & most powerful form of medicine or the slowest form of poison' and you can't get closer to the truth than that. After drinking good water, the next and most important thing you can do when it comes to food and nutrition is to commit to eating organic and I don't mean eating organic sometimes or selectively, but to commit to eating organic, period. Many people complain that the prices are too high for organic food or that there isn't an abundance of stores that carry organic products but these are only excuses as your health doesn't carry a price tag. It shouldn't be only that once someone becomes crippled with a life threatening disease that they are willing to change their lifestyle drastically as it's easiest and best to make those changes before one gets sick. Why are we okay with spending so much money to get better after falling ill but not willing to spend the money investing in our health before we get sick? Preventing disease is so much easier than curing it and why spend your life suffering until it's too late instead of taking back your power now and committing to doing whatever you need to to reach the perfect state of health? It makes sense to give up a few pleasures now so that we can live a longer and more fruitful life.

The demand for organic food is growing fast around the world and if there is a lack of organic produce in your local markets then make demands to fix that. It's up to the people to take back the power and change starts with us. If enough people request organic produce at a store then they will oblige and start carrying more and more organic produce so be the change, demand organic everywhere you go and question places that don't have it. The more organic produce we buy as a whole, the cheaper it will also become. There are numerous documentaries, articles, books and research papers that discuss the food industry, how dangerous eating a diet of GMO's is, how pesticides cause a staggering amount of disease in adults and children and you should educate yourself and know what you're eating. America is taking part in the biggest human experiment by consuming a diet that consists 90% of GMO's. Every time you eat out whether at a fast food take out or a fancy restaurant, unless it's an all organic menu, they are serving you food that isn't organic so why pay for something that will harm you?

The first issue with non organic produce is that they are usually GMO crops and they do not have the same nutrient content as organic produce. Why make all those salads, eat vegetables, juice or change your lifestyle when you're eating a product that only has a tenth of the nutrients it should? The second and more important reason of why eating GMO's is a bad choice for your health is that they go hand in hand with horrible long term side effects. There have been enough research studies that link GMO consumption with many forms of cancers, tumors as well as countless other damaging health risks. One of the biggest reasons we are seeing more and more people get sick at a younger age is due to a lifelong consumption of these GMO crops. Since GMO's were introduced to our markets in the 1980's, we've been consuming them without our permission or our knowledge and we are now starting to see the effects on a global scale. There is a drastic increase in tumors, cancers, rare diseases and younger and younger people are fighting illnesses that their grandparents maybe only saw in their old age. Sadly many people don't connect the two, thinking that food we consume cannot be responsible for such debilitating results. People are certain that the government wouldn't allow us to eat food that harmed us to such an extent but it's exactly this thinking that keeps us from being able to enforce a change in our food system and keeps letting the corruption to go on unnoticed. How can you NOT think that what you are consuming directly affects your health? Why would you take a risk with your body and your life when you only have one? You should be eating food that's natural at all times. If you do then even when you eat those food items that technically aren't the most healthy such as cheese, bread, pasta, pizza, cakes, they won't be nearly as bad for you as they will be made with organic ingredients.

Another thing that's great about buying organic is that you suddenly cut out all the dangerous pesticides and herbicides, many of which have been banned around the world but are still used here in the US and sprayed on practically everything. Agent orange is a poisonous toxic pesticide that is one of the most dangerous chemicals known to man and is recognized by the World health Organization as a carcinogen, confirmed to cause numerous cancers. It is also labeled by the American Academy of Medicine as a teratogen which causes birth defects. It has also been linked with Lymphoma, chronic lymphocytic leukemia, Hodgkin's disease, chloracne, prostate cancer, multiple myeloma, amyloidosis, Parkinson's disease, heart disease, hypertension, diabetes and cancers of larynx, lung, bronchia, trachea. Isn't it worthwhile to buy organic just to avoid that poison alone?

The reason organic costs more is that the produce is better and it's harder to grow crops without using chemicals. You should appreciate the farmer who chooses to grow organic and vote with your dollars as there is nothing more important than keeping your body healthy. There is nothing more important than keeping your family and children healthy. I'm sad when people complain about how expensive organic produce is but they are okay to spend $15 on a movie ticket or $30 on a face cream or $100 on a handbag. I think we need to prioritize what's most important and we can all agree that putting good quality, clean and nutritious food into our bodies is a top priority. So make a commitment to clean up your food intake, commit to buying only organic and commit to eating out at organic eateries. If there aren't any organic restaurants in your area then maybe it's best to stop eating out all together? Why pay expensive prices for restaurant food that's poisoning you? Look for organic cafes and restaurants and support those who are going out of their way to bring you healthy food.

When foods you love aren't available in the organic option make sure you speak with the store manager. Tell them that you want to see more organic produce and make suggestions for specific things you'd like. Nowadays with the internet you have no excuses so if there is something you want that your store doesn't carry then you can probably order it online in bulk. You can also order the ingredients and make it yourself. If there is no organic bread in your area, why not order some organic flour and yeast and make it a hobby to get into baking your own organic bread! If you don't have a good variety of organic vegetables maybe it's time to order organic seeds and start growing some vegetables at home. It's so much cheaper and so rewarding. You can start with just growing a few tomato plants in pots if you don't have a yard or look into turning your front lawn into a large vegetable garden, it's so easy and so cheap! I can't stress how important it is to avoid GMO's. If you can't afford organic or you don't see something in the organic option it's also good to look out for the NON GMO VERIFIED label that's popping up on a lot of items. They make sure that the ingredients are 100% non GMO and even though it's not fully organic it's still a huge step up from eating GMO's.

You should also look around your area and see if there are local farmers markets, small organic family farms, community gardens or co-ops. If there aren't any then maybe you can start one!

VEGETABLES:

Do you remember that food pyramid that you had to learn about in school that taught you about nutrition? Well it's time to forget it. Those food eating guides are incredibly out of date and also lack any real research. Humans do not thrive on an animal, grain and processed diet. Humans should be consuming a lot of vegetables and by a lot I all talking about 80% of every meal that you consume. The largest animals on the planet are herbivores and the biggest reason for why we can't seem to feel good is because we don't eat nearly the amount of vegetables that we need to truly fulfill our needs for nutrients. I believe we are herbivores too and it would be the most optimal to have a diet that consisted mainly of vegetables. Pretty much all the nutrients a human needs can be found in vegetables, you just need to make sure you eat more than just one carrot a day. The ultimate diet is 80% of raw or steamed vegetables with the rest of the 20% consisting of grains, nuts, legumes, dairy and fruits. Maybe that's not a possibility for you right now and that's okay but it's important to know what your diet should be if you wanted to eat your way to the perfect health. Without setting unrealistic goals and expectations for yourself, do your best by making sure that no matter what you committing to doing currently, to just include vegetables at every meal. You can do this at the very least and say that at every meal you will eat a raw or steamed vegetable and that you will also include all varieties. So if you absolutely cannot give up meat and you will still be having that burger for dinner, make a huge fresh salad and eat that first before even touching the burger. If you have to eat a pizza for lunch then snack on a few raw veggies first. Always have fresh organic vegetables in your fridge that you can grab and snack on anytime. This is a great way to retrain yourself, to eat the veggies FIRST and then other foods afterwards. This way you can fill yourself up a little so you can maybe eat less of the food that isn't that good for you. If you eat vegetables first and at every meal, like I described, you will ultimately be adding a massive amount of vegetables to your diet! Your absolute goal should be to consume fresh vegetables for 80% of your diet (canned vegetables do not count as fresh). I'm not saying that you have to do this overnight but slowly over time hopefully you can get to this ratio. There is no short cut around this so if you want to eat correctly start loving vegetables. Figure out ways you can make them delicious for you and include a variety of vegetables too. Don't get stuck with eating the same three vegetables and really explore all the varieties available, paying attention to what's in season. Make yummy organic veggie dips, vegetable bakes, grilled veggie sandwiches, BBQ veggie skewers and salads. Try to commit to eating one large salad every day. Fruit is good for you in many ways but please don't confuse fruit with vegetables as it's not the same thing. Fruit is a great thing to have as a snack but it will not take the place of vegetables. Often when I look at a clients diary of what they have been eating over a period of a week after I tell them to consume lots of vegetables, I'll often find that many think fruit and vegetables are the same thing. They are not and if you want to live a long and healthy life then start eating veggies of all sorts. After completing your detox, you should really attempt to eat a lot of vegetables, so make sure your fridge is stocked with them all the time. Buy lots of fresh vegetables and find great vegetarian recipes that you can experiment with. I would also highly recommend to keep drinking vegetable juices every day or as often as you can.

MORE OF THIS:

If you're eating 80% fresh vegetables then the other 20% should be made up of everything else that also serves your body in a good way such as nuts, fruit, seeds, legumes and grains. Make sure everything you purchase is unbleached, organic, untreated, untoasted and without unnecessary additives, salt or spices. You want to purchase the grain or nut in as close to it's natural state as possible. A roasted nut is not the same as a raw nut and the benefits a raw nut will give your body are endless! Also sprouting legumes, nuts and grains before eating unlocks the nutrients so try sprouting! It's so easy and requires little preparation. You can find instructions online for sprouting pretty much anything and all you'll need is some water and a jar!

Nuts and seeds - Make sure you are eating a variety of nuts and seeds. Don't get stuck always getting the almonds and never touching another nut, this is one of the biggest mistakes made with most people eating the same 10% of food items from their store. Try eating a handful of nuts every day and explore all of the varieties and always buy raw and untoasted nuts.

Whole grains - Wild rice, millet, quinoa, buckwheat, oats, bulgur, barley, rye, couscous. If you are buying bread, pizza dough, chips, pancake mix, crackers, cereal, pasta, make sure you don't constantly buy wheat products as this is what creates imbalance. Flour can be made from any grain so instead purchase products made from a variety of flours. You will see pasta made from not only wheat but buckwheat, rice, millet and quinoa! Don't ever purchase 'bleached' or 'white flour' products.

Legumes - Lentils, split peas, chickpeas, beans (explore all the bean varieties, we are always eating the same beans but there are so many).

Fresh fruit - The highest nutrient content comes from berries but always have fruit to snack on in your kitchen. Again make sure you buy a variety of fruit so don't get stuck eating the same thing over and over again.

Dried fruit – Dried fruit is alright in small amounts as a snack but I recommend avoiding it if you have a candida issue or get yeast infections often.

Dairy- The only thing I recommend from the dairy department in small and balanced amounts is raw goat milk and raw goat milk products. As much as cow milk is highly acidic, inflammatory and causes havoc in a human body, goat milk on the other hand, is highly alkaline, can be drank by people who are lactose intolerant and is not inflammatory at all, having the completely opposite effect. This only counts for goat milk that is raw which can be tough as that's illegal to sell in most states in the US but I have already seen it available in many co ops, shops and markets. You want to avoid pasteurized or homogenized milk as that process damages the milk and turns it acidic so if you're drinking goat milk but it's pasteurized then it's no good for you. There are some places that also sell raw goat cheese, raw goat yogurt and some other raw products so research around in your area, and see if you can find an Amish farm or someone with a goat who you can buy some raw milk from.

LESS OF THIS:

Now let's talk about the things that you should avoid as they don't do your body any good. Many people eat a diet that consists of nothing but the things I list below and this is exactly why they have been sick and also severely deficient in nutrients. Remember that changing your diet cannot be an overnight shift so don't try to eliminate everything at once and rather do it one item at a time. If you cannot quit eating something that is harmful then do your best to minimize the amount you eat or see if you can choose a healthier alternative. If you do eat it then please make sure to buy organic. Meat is bad enough in it's natural state when it's organic but it becomes pure poison when you add the hormones, chemicals, their GMO corn feed, steroids, antibiotics and from the time you consume it to the time it leaves your body, it does incredible damage to your body leaving a massive amount of carcinogens behind.

Meat - Consuming meat is just not good for anyone, period. The stories that humans have to consume meat to get proteins is nothing but a myth that has been disproven by hundreds of studies as well as millions of vegetarians around the world. The myth that certain people should eat meat because of their blood type is also nothing but a myth. The moment meat enters your body it turns poisonous and harms every single cell and as used to eating meat as you might be you have to address this huge factor if you want to be healthy. There are several amazing documentaries and research studies as well as books about how meat damages our cells, organs and tissues. We are similar in so many ways to herbivore animals and one of the most important similarities is that herbivores, like us, have very long intestines. All carnivorous animals without a doubt have short intestines and there is a reason for this difference that nature intended. The reason why meat eating animals have superbly short intestines is because meat turns toxic immediately after consumption, releasing numerous carcinogens, so the carnivore bodies are made to consume meat because they expel it out of their system very fast. When humans consume meat it has to travel for a very long time through our long intestines and it turns toxic while still inside us. Our jaws, teeth and stomach acids are also similar to herbivores and not equipped to consume meat. I won't even go into what happens to the meat when the animal is slaughtered and releases adrenaline and stress while they are dying, which is the meat that you consume afterwards. Ultimately I consider the consumption of meat one of the most toxic things on the menu. Still if you absolutely cannot completely cut meat out then try eating it less. Maybe you can cut down to eating it just once a week? Or maybe cut down to eating it just once a month? Maybe you can try changing meat to fish? I don't believe eating any red meat, poultry or fish is essential to us in any way so eat it as little as possible. Really try some alternatives that maybe you didn't consider before, there are so many amazing vegetarian options out there! Once you have a great veggie burger, I promise you that you will never look back.

Dairy products - As I mentioned already, cow products are extremely inflammatory and cause numerous illnesses. You can read the book called The China Study, which discusses one of the largest food health experiments ever done and it's effect on human health. The study was done over a 20 year period and it came down to one simple fact that consumption of animal products and meat is the single greatest cause of disease in humans. Cow milk in general is very unhealthy and this includes anything made with cow milk whether it's cheese, yogurt, ice cream or butter. There are great alternatives to cow milk such as raw goat milk as well rice and nut milks. Beware of the rice and nut milks sold in stores as a lot of those have been put through unnatural processes and are filled with many additives and preservatives. You can easily make your own nut milks at home, it's so simple and cheap! But whatever you do stop consuming cow milk and cow milk products.

Junk foods - So you love going to the local burger shop and getting that 5.99 meal that tastes so good but do you ever wonder what it's made of and how much damage it's doing to your body? Maybe you prefer not to think about it or you block it out so you don't feel guilty but you have to come to a realization that if you keep consuming junk food, then eventually you will have a broken body. You have to make a choice that no matter the cravings, no matter the situation, you will be aware of every bite that goes in and you will choose what's best for you. I don't have to explain why junk food is bad or what toxic chemicals and ingredients are used to make it and you know that the reason it's so cheap is because they don't use real food ingredients. Avoid junk food at all costs and if you do eat out try to look for organic places or at least healthier options. You can practically find everything you love in a healthier and better alternative so just say no to junk food. There is no way getting around this, you need to re-train your brain to not liking this stuff. Everyone has those late night cravings after a long night out or a long day at the office and you need to find a way to satisfy those cravings using natural foods that don't harm you. Choose some organic quick cook meals that can be sitting in your pantry or freezer that you can eat in times when you are tempted to buy junk food. I keep some organic boxes of mac 'n cheese in my kitchen for those times and it takes me 10 minutes to have it ready, and although it's not the healthiest option, it's so much better than junk food.

So next time you go shopping make sure you stock up on something that can fill that craving for junk food.

Processed foods - If you're eating something that has the shelf life of five years then how can that be the fuel you choose to put into your body expecting it to thrive, feel good and make you happy? What you put in is what you get out. With processed food you are either eating empty calories with no benefits whatsoever or even worse, you're eating toxic food that causes much harm. If it's packaged in a box with a best before date of a year from now then it cannot be LIVE food. If you want to feel alive then you have to eat alive food. Food that can sit in a box for years is not alive or filled with so much preservatives that it's best to avoid it. Try to get further away from the processed stuff. Attempt to cut anything that sits on a shelf and replace it with a live food.

Sugar – As a society we consume a scary amount of sugar. Sugar is added to everything and you might not even be aware of how much sugar you consume on a daily basis. Studies have found that the same part of the brain lights up when you eat sugar as when you take cocaine and sugar is highly addictive and detrimental to your health. All tumors, growths and cancers feed on sugars and if you eat sugar daily and in large amounts then you're directly poisoning yourself. Natural sugar that's found in fruit is different as it's attached to fiber so our bodies process is differently but the sugar that comes extracted, bleached and processed is no good. It's okay to eat sweets or sugar in moderation and important to use healthier alternatives like agave, molasses, honey, coconut sugar or maple syrup but one has to be in balance. Never consume more than one treat at a time and try to go a day without sugar, none in your coffee, none on your cereal, no snacks or sweets and nothing that has sugar as an ingredient. You will see how difficult this is and you might even get a sugar withdrawal. Be aware and know what you're consuming. I have a rule in my house that if I want snacks or sweets that I have to make my own from scratch, so when I have to get up and go bake a batch of cookies it sure makes me think twice whether I want cookies at all.

White flour foods - Anything that is white is no good as that means it's been bleached and put through a refining processing that strips the grain of any potential nutrients it had before. When you are consuming wheat products, which should be in moderation anyway, make sure you always purchase whole wheat. Whole wheat pasta, whole wheat bread, whole wheat pizza, whole wheat crackers.... Check the ingredients and anything that says white flour, bleached flour, flour, refined flour, wheat flour usually means it's been stripped of the top layer of the wheat grain which does no good for you. A huge difference between white flour and whole flour is the fiber content. Fiber is essential to numerous body functions like being regular with your bowel movements, lowering blood cholesterol and weight loss and in white flour the fiber rich part of the grain has been stripped and removed leaving hardly any fiber. Another thing that's affected is the blood sugar levels as eating whole wheat absorbs slowly preventing blood sugar spikes and crashes leaving you satisfied for longer after your meal. Also whole flour is rich in folate, riboflavin, vitamins B1, B3 and B5 while white flour is stripped of all it's vitamins leaving you with nothing.

Sodas & juice - drinking any sugary drinks is just a missed chance of drinking water which is liquid gold for your body, instead you are choosing to drink liquid sugars with other potentially harmful additives and chemicals. I don't need to explain why sodas are bad for you and you need to eliminate them from your life completely. As much as sodas are bad, most other sugary drinks that are disguised as healthy like ice teas, vitamin waters, processed and pasteurized vegetable and fruit juices are no good either. You'll notice that after giving them up for a period of time that you will not enjoy their taste or flavor any more so it's just about getting it out of your system. There are several drinks on the market that are healthy and that's the ones that have no added sugar, have only a few ingredients on the label and all are things you know with no long names of chemicals. Mostly it would be best to get used to drinking water all the time when you're thirsty. Herbal teas that are organic are great too and so is coconut water. And have you ever made home made lemonade?? It's the best.

RULES OF HEALTHY EATING:

Close to the source

You should always have this in mind when choosing which products to put in your body - 'how close to the source is it?' When you question whether something is healthy or not then just ask yourself how close to the source it is. If you take any healthy food item and you let it sit on a plate for a month it will turn rotten, so if you purchase something in a box and it's good for a year and will stay good once opened for a month then how is that possibly good for you? Also if it was picked, made and packaged months ago how is it possible that this will still have any nutrients in it? So you truly want to get closer to the source… eat food that's fresh, was recently plucked from the earth, eat food that is ALIVE. Dead food does nothing for you or your health. Dead food comes in bags, boxes and plastic. If you follow this rule and you eat at least 80% of your food close to the source then you will make huge strides towards a healthier you.

Cooking

When you're cooking food please try to avoid frying or boiling if you can. Frying and boiling food kills it and kills the nutrients. If you must fry then do so for as short a time as you can and use organic coconut oil as it doesn't heat up as much as other oils and it's hugely beneficial for you. Steaming or baking are best methods of cooking and not as damaging. When steaming vegetables it's best to leave the vegetables a little on the crispy side so don't overdo it. I of course recommend never ever using the microwave and if you are making something requiring frying you can always steam it first then flash fry quick at the end just to give it a little more flavor.

Chewing

Well this is an overlooked benefit and a huge one. Eating in a rush and not chewing properly is a waste even if you're eating the healthiest food there is as it amounts to you losing half the nutrients you are eating. When you swallow without chewing properly, the body cannot assimilate any of the nutrients from the food. Digestion begins in the mouth and chewing every bite well is very important. If you chew your food well you will be giving your body much more benefits so commit to slowing down and really being aware of how you're eating.

Relaxed eating

Eating is an important part of life and although we are busy and things are constantly happening around us, we need to create a moment to eat without too many distractions. It is difficult to do this when there doesn't seem to be enough hours in the day to get everything done but it's vital that when you are consuming food that you are not doing anything else so that your body and mind can focus on this activity and so you can get the best out of it. Also you should feel good when eating as if you're upset or angry then you're bound to have trouble digesting. You need to be fully relaxed, forget everything else and just eat, slowly, deliberately and with full awareness. Truly taste the food, feel the consistency of it on your tongue and have positive thoughts and feelings about the food. It's also a placebo effect, if you're telling your body that this food you're eating tastes horrible and you hate it, your body will hate it too. Enjoy the food, feel good and your body will enjoy it too.

Summary

Maybe at this point you are feeling overwhelmed by all this information and wondering if you can change your lifestyle this much at all. Maybe you're questioning whether you can really eat an 80% all vegetable diet but I want you to know that it's normal to have fears and doubts but that you have no choice and must push on if you want to get healthy. Take it one step at a time and go as slow as you need to. When you are making huge lifestyle changes you must have patience with yourself and know that even small steps forward are steps nonetheless. Nobody is saying you have to make all the changes overnight as that's unrealistic and utterly impossible so do what you can. Improve your diet little by little one day at a time. So if you ate junk food every day, see if you can just eat it once a week, if you eat meat every day see if you can eat it once a week.... If you cannot quit eating your favorite candy then eat a huge salad first and then reward yourself later by allowing yourself to have that candy. It's all about balance and slowly change your habits one by one. A good rule is to incorporate something new every week so you could start with the first week of swapping all your meat to fresh non processed meats and then the second week you try to cut down on sugar and so on. It's all about what you can do for yourself, don't be harsh on your progress, we are all different and go at difference paces but know that every little bit counts and every thing you put in your body you're either nourishing it or poisoning it.

EXAMPLE OF GOOD DIET:

Breakfast ideas

(select a few and remember that breakfast = break-fast, it's just a time for us to break the short fast we did while sleeping so don't overeat and have a small breakfast, throw out that myth that a large breakfast is a good breakfast.)

* Herbal tea or Fresh vegetable juice

* Select raw vegetables with organic dip or salad dressing

* Fresh fruit

* Granola & raw goat milk / yogurt

* Buckwheat porridge

* Whole grain toast & coconut oil

* Boiled egg

Lunch ideas:

*Salad (lettuce/spinach/arugula, tomato, cucumber, carrot….) topped with your favorite organic salad dressing or coconut/olive oil and topping like pumpkin seeds, raw goat cheese, nuts and sprouts.

* Sandwich with whole grain bread or wrap with whole grain tortilla stacked with any one or few fresh vegetables (cucumber, grated carrot, cabbage, spinach, arugula) topped with avocado, flax seeds, pumpkin seeds, raw goat cheese or nut cheese or hummus

* Home made salsa & guacamole with healthy chips (non GMO)

* Home made vegetable soup

Dinner ideas:

* Home made veggie burger on a sprouted whole grain bun with a salad and mashed potato

* Steamed vegetables with some grains (wild rice / quinoa / lentils) with pesto and sun dried tomatoes

* Vegetable bake (select vegetables drilled with oil, spices and goat cheese baked in a bowl)

* Vegetarian chili

Dessert ideas:

* Home baked banana bread

* Avocado chocolate pudding

* Nuts & honey mix

* Coconut milk ice cream with raspberries

Snacks:

Always have snacks on the go so you don't starve and then go silly with eating the wrong stuff. Carry a small glass container with your favorite nuts, dried berries (cranberries/goji), fresh vegetables like baby carrots, fresh or dried fruit.

* * *

THE EXERCISE:

This chapter has a lot of exercises so take it a day at a time to make sure you complete them all before you move on to the next part, even if it takes a month to complete them all! Do what you can today and then as you have free time on the upcoming days keep working on the next exercise. Be proud of yourself and give yourself some credit.

* Get healthy water, weather it's ordering spring water or buying a quality filtration system. Make a commitment to never drink from plastic bottles and purchase an aluminum water bottle that you can use to take water with you on the go every day. If you can't afford an expensive water filtration system for the home or you are waiting to get your spring water delivered in a week, buy a family sized cheap water filter in a local store for the mean time.

* Look up farmers markets are in your area and make a list of them to put up on your fridge so you remember to visit them. Also look up any co-ops and community gardens.

* Make a commitment to buy organic or Non Gmo as much as you can when shopping also make a commitment to avoid non organic eating out. Research whether there are any organic or healthier eating out options in your area and make a list of them. Yes this will be one of the most

difficult and financially painful processes but this is the part that truly matters.

* Commit to grow. Find a space in your yard or plant some stuff in pots indoors, even if it's a small herb garden or a few tomato plants. Grow some of your own food and start right now by ordering some organic heirloom seeds that are not GMO today.

* Make a list of all the vegetables that exist that are available for purchase. Put that list on your fridge with space next to the list and check off three vegetables a day starting today that you eat. Do not move onto repeating buying the same vegetables until you've consumed all the vegetables at some point. Once done then start all over again. This is called eating a VARIETY of vitamins and nutrients.

* Make a list of two columns, one is MORE OF THIS and the other is LESS OF THIS. Write all the things that fall under each one. Decide what you are willing to cut out completely from the 'less of this' category. Make a note next to things that you cannot completely cut out and commit to eating them less often. Make a deal with yourself on what you will sacrifice for your health and be specific. Cross out whatever you are cutting out and put this list up on your fridge as well.

* Commit to writing a meal journal for a minimum of a week so you can assess what you are eating. Every night

before bedtime write down what you ate that day so you can review it. This will allow you to see whether you are reaching the 80/20 vegetables ratio. It helps to visually see what you are consuming. After keeping the journal for a while, read it and ask yourself whether you are feeding your body well and if it's the best you can do.

* Purchase a vegetable steamer and commit to steaming vegetables when cooking instead of frying or boiling.

* Purchase a vegetable juicer and commit to drinking vegetable juices as often as you can but at least three times a week, preferably daily. If you cannot commit to drinking vegetable juices then consider getting a blender instead and make smoothies.

* Find and save healthy recipes that look appetizing that are made with organic and vegetarian ingredients and commit to making at least one thing a week even if you've never cooked before.

STEP FOUR

Movement

Of all the things I struggle with, I am one of those who find it difficult to exercise just as much as the next person. It seems that it's always a struggle to keep it up as well as finding the time to do it. When you finally do have some free time it's much easier to use that time to relax and unwind instead of running on a treadmill. Back in the day people exercised naturally without having to plan the activity but since our current lifestyles don't include farming in the fields or walking for miles to the store, we need to put emphasis on exercise and even if organized exercise isn't something you can commit you, you need to at least involve some sort of movement in your life every single day without fail.

Fitting in exercise into the whole day

I have a rule about sitting for too long and I always check my watch and when it's been an hour and I've been stagnant, I jump up and I do something to move my body. It could be anything from some yoga stretches, touching my toes, jumping around to music or just going for a quick walk around the block. Of course if you're at the office this might not be possible without drawing some strange looks from co-workers but you could still do some leg stretches, flex your feet and circle them, circle your head and stretch your neck. You might even get away with standing up and doing some stretches. It's about incorporating it whenever you can and the reality is there are many ways to incorporate it in all the time. Anywhere there is an elevator there also are.... stairs! You should always choose to forgo the elevator and take the stairs. Are you driving somewhere that's only three blocks away? Leave the car and go walking, make it an adventure. I also made a rule about watching TV as that's already such a dead brain activity so when I watch TV, I pull out my mini trampoline that I have in my room and I bounce around on it as much as I can while I'm watching. Trampolines also have this magical effect on your brain which helps regulate moods and help with depression. For every 30 minutes of TV, I commit to jumping on the trampoline for 10 minutes. Make little agreements with yourself about how you'll start moving around and it doesn't have to be an organized class or a set time. It's about incorporating movement into every single activity you're doing throughout your day. Just because you don't have the time to do a full hour gym class, that's not an excuse and you can still do a little bit of here and there so put on your favorite album when you get home from work and dance around in your living room to get your blood pumping. Even buying a jump rope and jumping for a few minutes will do wonders! Of course doing an hour of exercise every day would be truly wonderful but most people make the mistake of thinking that if they cannot do an hour of exercise that they'll skip it all together, when you could literally do as little as a five minutes a day.

Getting your sweat on

One of the main ways to measure your exercise level and whether you're doing a good job is by the sweat. Sweating is a great way that your body can flush out toxins and it should be your goal to get your body to sweat every day. Besides taking stairs or doing stretches, doing cardio style exercise at least three times a week is vital so you need to implement this through whatever cardio exercise you enjoy. I always recommend finding something fun to do so you're not bored or having to absolutely despise the times you have set aside for exercise. Do some research and find something in your area that maybe you haven't tried before, maybe a dance class or a community night hikes. It doesn't always have to be the same thing and it's about being creative and thinking of ways you can get your exercise in by also having fun and joining in with others who are doing the same. Commit to finding ways to sweat as your skin is the largest organ and if you made a commitment to get sweating every day you would find to have done a large amount of detoxing after 30 days so make a point to get sweating no matter how you get there!

Nature

Human beings need nature as much as animals do and it does every single thing necessary to balance and ground every cell and hormone in our bodies. Nowadays most people spend all their time indoors and hardly spend any time outside which is vital to being healthy. Sunshine, fresh air and time spent in nature is something that can not only renew your soul but has a multitude of health benefits. If you can combine spending time outside with exercise then it's even better. Call up a friend and ask them to play a weekly game of tennis or organize a group hike. Spend your weekends away from your house and the city whether it's camping in the forest or yoga in the park. It's absolutely important that you spend as much time outside as you can and don't only spend time outside but actually get grounded by getting your feet on the grass, sand or dirt and touching trees and so on. Being close with nature will do so much for you health wise. If you have a dog then head out on a long day hike and get them some exercise as well as yourself or at least make a commitment to walk them around the block every evening. Growing your own vegetables is a great way to get some healthy and affordable fresh produce into your kitchen and it's a way to get some exercise too so I urge you plant a garden. Basically do whatever it takes to spend as much time outdoors and make sure that from a typical day you're getting a dose of being outside for at least half an hour.

* * *

THE EXERCISE:

Make the following agreements to help bring movement into your life:

* For every hour of sitting I'll stand up and make an effort to do some stretches or movement. (Use an alarm as a reminder if you need to!)

* I will not take the elevator and use the stairs instead.

* If the drive is less than 5 minutes, I will choose to walk.

* I will plan at least one activity outdoors every week.

* While watching TV I will do some sort of exercise for a part of it whether it's stretching or jumping jacks.

* I will get my body sweating at least three times a week through fun organized exercise classes or groups.

* I am going to purchase one item that will help me to exercise (trampoline, jump rope, bike, tennis racket)

MAKE A COMMITMENT TO MAKE MOVEMENT AND THE OUTDOORS A PART OF YOUR LIFE.

STEP FIVE

Cutting the negative

We are now done with the physical aspects of health and are moving onto the mental aspects. You should carry on with many of the exercises and commitments discussed in previous chapters and keep improving your life day by day and we will now start to focus on some of the ways you are harming your life by your thoughts and behavior.

One of the main things that separate us from animals is that we have the capacity to think and create thought patterns. One of the ways that we do damage to ourselves is by living in a fictional space in our heads where we've created thought patterns that are destructive and serve no purpose. A wild mind thinking chronically negative thoughts will affect every part of your life from your relationships, to your physical health, your work and your mental state. Of course we are all made a little different, some people are naturally more positive and up beat and others naturally pessimistic, some are pretty relaxed about everything and others much more nervous, some handle stress really well and others struggle with it, but one thing is for certain and that is that every person, no matter what they are like currently, will benefit from reformatting their mind. Remember that the point of these exercises isn't to judge yourself, measure yourself against others, beat yourself up or spend extended periods of time analyzing why you are this or that way but rather spend your energy on strengthening your skills, gaining control of the thoughts and steering them towards a positive space. I've broken the chapter down into smaller sections but ultimately they all boil down to the main theme of 'BE POSITIVE: Think positive, Speak positive, Act positive'. Even if none of your actual circumstances change, there is a huge difference between living in a positive space and living in a negative space which has dramatic results on how you feel and how your body functions. Just like everything else in life, lasting change and real benefits do not come easily but are achieved with hard work, commitment and daily practice.

Cut out the negative thoughts

Currently there is scientific evidence that your thoughts and your mental state affects your entire physical body. Every time you have a negative thought whether it's about someone or something, it affects you, showing up on a brain scanning device to disrupt electric signal functions in the brain which as we know is what's happening on a major level during depression and mood disorders and it slows down your brain coordinator, making it difficult to process new thoughts or problem solve. It also decreases activity in your cerebellum, which is responsible for motor control and cognitive function and impacts your left temporal lobe, which affects mood, memory and impulse control. And that's just the brain! Speaking negatively has the same effect if not more damaging. Of course being negative also raises your stress levels which is connected to heart problems, high blood pressure, depression, anxiety, diabetes, skin conditions, asthma, arthritis and headaches. Another thing that living in a negative space does to impact your life in a bad way is that it also takes you away from the present and the ability to enjoy whatever it is you are doing in that moment. You cannot fully be enjoying a movie, hanging out with a friend or eating a delicious dinner if you're cycling over negative thoughts at the same time. You also are not fun to be around and this energy spreads to others and is seen and felt much more than you think. Nobody will say that having chronic pessimistic thoughts or speaking negatively brings them joy, peace or happiness. Also the excuse that you cannot be in a positive place because you have so many problems or that life is giving you a raw deal is just that, an excuse. No matter how bad your life is or how many problems you have, you will benefit a great deal by moving yourself into a positive mental space. The circumstances do not and should not rule how you are feeling as the only time you will have no problems is when your life is over so accept that you will always be dealing with things and accept responsibility for your wild mind. It's also a downward spiral as a negative thought will turn into a negative vocalization which will progress into negative action and if you really become aware and start to notice this pattern, you will see that that's the reason many bad things happen all at once. We are often responsible for the negativity we create in our own lives.

Changing any habit whether it's smoking cigarettes or eating candy is hard enough but changing your thought patterns is much more difficult as it's not a physical change that you can see or touch so it's really easy to keep slipping back to our old ways of thinking without even noticing it. The idea is to practice this on a daily basis, just like learning to play an instrument or a language. You need to commit to doing this and doing it every single day.

The first step will be becoming so aware that you are able to notice your thoughts throughout the day while you go on with your activities. The second step will be to stop the thoughts that are negative as soon as you notice them, eliminate them or replace them with a positive one. At first this might seem like a full time job and really tedious but everything learned has to be un-learned so be patient. When you first start attempting this you will realize how little control your have over your own mind and what a wild animal it actually is! It's like it has a mind of it's own and doesn't belong to you which can be a scary realization as you should have control over every function in your own body especially your thinking. The goal will be to stay on course with the exercise and eventually to reach a point when you go through your entire day avoiding all negative thinking or speaking but before you get there it will test you over and over and over again. I mainly speak about and concern myself with negative thinking as that's where the negativity begins at but it's anything negative that should be cut out so speaking negatively about yourself, others and life in general is just as bad. Also if you are catching yourself doing negative things like hurting someone, screaming at the dog, stealing or manipulating someones life then obviously you missed countless negative thoughts that you should have caught before it reached the action stage.

You might do really well for one or two days and then you wake up on the third wake up really late for work, the cat peed on your rug, you burn yourself with hot coffee in the kitchen, rushing out you notice that someone vandalized your mailbox, then on the way you quickly pop into the bank where you see a really long line and while waiting someone cuts in line and finally you give in and fall into that negative space, just festering judgment and contempt for this total stranger at the bank, all the while stressing, raising your heart rate and throwing you completely out of your mental balance. Afterwards you rush out of the bank, get in your car and reverse out of the parking space forgetting to check both sides and you smash into a car that you didn't see. Now this is a perfect example of what happens when we let ourselves back into the negative space. Had we had enough awareness to notice the negative thought pattern while still in line at the bank, we could have replaced it with a positive thought, possibly coming up with reasons for why that person had to cut in line and what emergency they might have had, choosing to come from a place of understanding and compassion which might have changed our circumstances. Remember that you will have set backs all the time and you just simply need to notice it and get back on track. Each day and each moment will be a challenge but the goal is to stay patient and stick to it. Just like you can't learn a language overnight, you can't change your mind overnight. It will take patience and work but the longer you practice, the easier it will get. Remind yourself that for *your health* it's important to stay calm and to stay positive no matter what is happening around you. Being negative in thought, words or actions will not make your circumstances better and in fact it's pretty much always guaranteed to make the circumstances worse.

<u>Live in the present</u>

Another form of toxic mind pattern is being constantly stuck in the past or stuck in the future and this is another difficult one to stop doing but it completely robs you of the present moment just the same. Only a small portion of times when we are thinking about the past or the future are useful to us and most of the time it's doing this that causes more anxiety, worry and suffering.

If you added up all the time you have spent worrying about what will happen in the future, how many days do you think that would add up to? Probably not days but months or years, time that you cannot get back no matter how much you wish to. Thinking over and over about stressful upcoming events or situations and playing out all the possible ways it could turn out is plain insanity but it's an insanity that almost everyone is guilty of. Again this serves no purpose and you cannot predict the future so this cycling over something that hasn't happened yet is pointless. Of course some thoughts about the future will occur, but I'm speaking of a habitual constant worrying that never stops. Worrying about the future does not make the outcome different nor does it allow you to control the situations better but only takes away from you enjoying the current moment.

And how much time have you spent day dreaming about the past? Thinking about what you should have done, how you should have answered or reacted, how you would have turned out had your parents not done this or that, going over and over things that have happened that you can never change, mistakes you made, regrets, all of this is okay to reflect upon for a minute but being in an obsessive mind cycle of constantly not being able to let go of the past is not serving you in any positive way.

Not living in the current moment is something that almost everyone suffers from but people are waking up to the reality that without letting go of the past and without letting go of worrying about the future, you cannot find peace or happiness in the now and the now is all that you have a guarantee of. People who suffer from insomnia are often riddled with either spending time mowing over the events of the day and what happened or stressing about tomorrow. Over thinking, obsessing, worrying and analyzing is an addiction of the mind as the mind always wants to feel busy, it wants to be going at full speed and it's easier for the mind to be elsewhere than in the present moment. This is a cycle that you go into day after day and it's not going to change in one second just because you read this chapter. You need to make a commitment to change the patterns and cycles of the brain. If you can achieve this, even little by little, you will notice a shift not only in the way you are feeling but you will suddenly see small changes occurring in every aspect of your life. We can never fully be 100% in the moment if we are somewhere else in our thoughts. So maybe you're eating dinner with your loved one that you could be more present with which would be a completely different experience all together or maybe you're with a friend spending time with them, or you're walking your dog or working on a project... but no matter what it is you're doing, if you mind is not in present then you're missing out. This is a habit that most people end up in their whole lives and are never ever in the current moment which is truly sad.

Of course small amounts of time can be spent remembering something or planning something in the future but even that must be kept constructive and to a minimum. There is a clear difference between thinking of the past/future in a constructive way and a destructive way. Make sure you understand the difference. It's okay to reflect or to browse over upcoming events but doing so obsessively and in a negative manner is not only useless but bad for your health. For example, this is constructive thinking 'well that did not go well because of the choices I made, but next time I will do this and that differently and I look forward to trying this again with a better outcome', instead of the destructive thinking, 'I can't believe this happened, this is why I don't do anything, because everything I try fails. I'm a real loser and life never gives me a break.' What's the point in having negative thoughts about something in the past that you can't change? You never know when it will be the last moment of your life, you also don't know when it will be the last moment of life for anyone else so imagine your loved one passing away and you realize that your last exchange was you spending hours complaining about a proposal that could have gone better.

Less stuff, more living

Addiction to having more material possessions, earning more money, buying a bigger house, more clothing, a better car and so on is a serious addiction that only leads down a road of unhappiness. You do not have to prove anything to anybody, especially not yourself. Owning more things and achieving more will not bring you happiness and you need to break away from such thinking. We often trick ourselves into believing we really need this thing or that thing when we truly only need a few basic things like food to eat, a roof over our heads and maybe a few comfort items. The real things in life that actually matter are not at all the material things but the experiences, the relationships and so on. Let go of the addiction of needing new things. Let go of the addiction of wanting new things. Don't make it a habit of teaching your children that they will be rewarded with material possessions and don't use material stuff to show love either. The best gifts to loved ones shouldn't be material things! Let go of the addiction to always replace material possessions that don't need replacing and constantly ask yourself whether you really really need this item or if it's just the consumer mind talking.

Stress and the yo yo of life

Here is a guarantee for you - life has it's ups and downs, all the time, without fail and hardly ever are you just standing still, with nothing going on having a completely stable experience. The illusion that one day you will reach this plateau in your life when there will no longer be ups or downs is delusional. No matter how wise you get, what successes you achieve, who you marry or how much money you make, life will always be throwing you curve balls and you should see this as an exciting principle of life instead of fearing or trying to avoid it. See life as an adventure that's always filled with change, spontaneity and excitement and you can accept that in a positive way and stop expecting things to finally "settle down". Take it with the good and the bad and accept it, go with the flow of life. We have an addiction to a thinking that once we fix all our problems we currently have, then we can relax and enjoy life, while we all know that this will never happen as new issues arrive daily. Accepting that life is always going to be a roller coaster ride can actually lead you to understand that you do not need to be so emotionally affected by it and instead find a way to be stable and stress free. To over react to every event that takes place or to bottle up stress is not only tiring mentally but it's tiring on a physical level as well. As much as most of us spend our days stressing, I doubt anyone would argue that stress somehow benefits your life. Originally this was a natural reaction that served our ancestors in life-threatening situations awakening the fight or flight censor but in the current day and age, we stress mainly out of habit. Of course some minor stress will happen at times when we are meant to perform, whether at a work presentation or at a risky outdoor activity but I'm speaking more of the underlying chronic stress that most of us go through daily with no end in sight. Stress is linked to all major physical illnesses and cells in the body have been shown to act completely erratically when under stress and long term chronic stress has major health hazzards. Everything physically is affected the moment you begin stressing with stress hormones slowing the stomach, interfering with digestive function, it causes headaches, increases your heart rate and blood pressure, raises cholesterol levels raising your risk of heart attacks and strokes. Stress weakens your immune system dramatically and slows any healing processes in the body. It also causes you to crave fats and carbohydrates adding to weight gain and weight gain that's caused by stress usually focuses on belly fat which raises risks of heart disease and diabetes. It can create a constant state of tension and anxiety on your mental state which can lead to depression, migraines and insomnia. The way to deal with any issues that arise that you feel stress you out, is to address the issue immediately and logically without drawing it out into a lengthy and painful process. Do not drive yourself mental with any issue and remind yourself that everything will pass in due time. Logically when you feel stressed or even before you get to that point, know that you either *CAN* do something about it, or you *CANNOT*. Without being emotional, irrational or stressed out, make a constructive decision on what you can do and then do it. Don't spend days, weeks or months torturing yourself, just decide, take action and move on with your life productively. No need for all the pessimistic and dramatic judgments or thoughts, just productive action. If there is nothing you can do about it then you have to accept it and move on and don't waste even one more minute thinking about it. Often you see people over reacting or stressing about things that are not at all important in the big picture or stressing about things that they have zero control over and both of those can lead to utter madness. Learn to grow into a mentally strong person. We admire people who are physically strong but being mentally strong is even more important. No matter what issue arises or how your life falls apart, remind yourself that eventually things will be normal again or you will adapt to the issue.

If you are a person who would like to stop stressing but find it incredibly difficult then you need to figure out methods that work for you to relieve stress. Implement ways to de-stress yourself and actually use them at times when you feel yourself starting to go into a loop of stress.

Every time you feel the stress eating away at you, have a plan of action in place that can allow you to release the stress. It can be a breathing exercise, getting a boxing bag and gloves that you hang up in your garage that you go at when stressed, calling a friend, doing arts & crafts, doing a visualization exercise, jogging, putting on soothing music and so on. Figure out something specific that helps you to de-stress and then immediately jump on doing that when you feel out of control stress-wise.

Also practicing silent sitting meditation daily calms the mind and is one of the best ways to cure yourself of chronic stress. Of course meditation might not be for everyone and for some it's near impossible but I do believe it helps everyone when used correctly and often. In the beginning meditation can seem like pulling teeth but it's like anything else in life and with practice, little by little you'll start feeling less pain and more results. Once learned it can be used anywhere from a quiet corner of your tranquil home to your car in the middle of a busy city street. It's a way for us to shut down our brain and give everything a little break. As much as we give our bodies rest when sleeping, our brains never get a break, being forced to run at full speed from the day we were born until death so meditation is that little vacation for your mental processing plant that gives instant relief for stress and promotes a feeling of well being and happiness.

BE positive, BE centered, BE you

Have you met one of those people who just walk into the room and immediately you're lit up by their energy? Suddenly everyone notices them, is drawn to them, wants to be their friend and speak to them. When you do speak to them you feel energized and elated. They carry an energy that is calm, positive, peaceful and compassionate. The energy spreads to everyone around them and that's the kind of person that you should try to become. If you compare that person to someone who has a sour look on their face, from the moment you see them seem incredibly upset, bored and uninterested in everything. Everything that comes out of their mouth is a complaint, a judgment of someone or just plain negative. Imagine they find something wrong with everything, they seem angry, jealous, unfulfilled and generally unfriendly. Now which person would you rather spend your time around? Which person do you wish you could be? You can choose to be the person who everyone wants to be around, you can choose to be the person that's a delight and not a weight.

*   *   *

THE EXERCISE:

I want you to take your time with these exercises. Don't rush through them as it's supposed to break your bad habits. Spend each day focussed and committed.

FIRST WEEK: Changing the negative.

For a whole week after reading this chapter you will try to cut the negative from your life. Put up little notes and reminders for yourself to start being aware of your thoughts all around the house, car, workplace and so on. Without reminders it will be difficult to remember so if you need to, set an alarm to go off on your cellphone every 30 minutes, but stay aware of your thoughts.

Examples of great reminders to put around your home:

* What are you thinking NOW?

* Are you being POSITIVE or NEGATIVE?

* What energy are you spreading?

The exercise is to spend the week noticing whether you are in a positive or negative space. Try to ask yourself and notice this throughout the day, every hour, every minute or every second. Try to go through an entire day being and thinking positive with as little negativity or complaints as you can. You especially need to focus on this when things go wrong, when people are rude or when things don't turn out the way you wished them to. Negative thoughts or feelings are all harmful whether it's about yourself, about others or about a situation. Notice every time you speak to someone whether you are saying positive or negative things and of course making a joke or explaining what happened is alright but make sure it's not constantly the sarcasm, judgement or depression talking.

Here are list of negative thoughts that don't serve us in a good way -

* I'm such a loser, I can't do anything right.

* She annoys me so much, what a total idiot.

* My life is horrible, nothing ever works out.

* I'm so broke, next month will be impossible.

* Things never seem to work out for me

* I won't even bother doing that as it'll probably fail.

* Nobody likes me anyway

* There is no point in trying at all

* I hate life / I hate him / I hate myself.

* Everyone Is so stupid.

* Why am I so unlucky.

The difference between someone happy and unhappy isn't outside circumstance at all but it's how they look at things. If you can become aware of your thoughts and start eliminating negative thought patterns then you will feel better. Initially the trick is to simply notice every time you're having a negative thought and immediately over ride it with a positive one so keep reminding yourself to be aware and notice negative thoughts and eradicate them or replace them with a positive. Also watch when you speak, are you always complaining? Are you spreading your negativity to others vocally? Are you doing negative actions towards others? Notice and keep replacing everything with a positive even if it's difficult to think of a positive when something has gone wrong, try really hard and keep doing this until it becomes more natural.

SECOND WEEK: Live in the present.

The second week is going to be focussed on being in the present. You should still keep trying to cut the negative, but just add this to the plate. It's now time to practice being aware of your thoughts and see whether you are mostly in the present moment or constantly stuck in the past or the future. Do not spend time going over and over something that has already taken place and also do not spend time worrying about how something might happen in the future. Give up that need to control everything and just allow things to unfold as they are. Whatever happened in the past, let it go. Whatever will happen in the future, let it be. Any thoughts that begin with 'I can't believe that.....' or 'If only I had done....' or 'I'm so worried that he just won't....' or 'I wish I knew.....' are all living in past or present. BE mindful, enjoy the things you are doing NOW and live life NOW instead of time traveling in your mind.

Keep practicing all week to catch yourself whenever you're not in the present and then bring your thoughts back to the present moment. Also make sure you are not verbalizing being in the past or the future as well. For example if you have spent a lengthy amount of time speaking to a loved one, friend or relative about a certain topic that is in the past/future that isn't productive and just simply fretting or fussing negatively then stop and talk about something else. Remember to try be the person everyone wants to be around and although it's okay to confide and share things with people around you, if you catch yourself going over and over the same thing that you have no control over then it's probably a sign that you should stop and move on.

THIRD WEEK: Manage stress

Although stress is often called the silent killer, combatting stress isn't as easy as one might imagine. This week really try to focus on eliminating stress from your life. Of course eating correctly and exercise help as well as meditation which is discussed in the next chapter but directly addressing the issues you are stressing about is a good idea as well.

I want you to think of some stress relieving techniques that could work for you and write them down in a book or journal. Try them out one by one and see which work and which do not. Be proactive about it and remember to actually use them. It's important to have something to DO actively when stress overcomes you.

Then dedicate a good amount of time to sit and write down a list of current issues that are stressing you out no matter if they are big or small. Take the time to really think about all areas of your life and be honest with yourself. Anything that can potentially be adding to your stress levels even in the slightest should be noted. Once you are done writing the list then address each issue asking whether you CAN or CANNOT do something about it. If you can do something about it, write down a solution for each one. If you cannot do anything about it then spend a few minutes accepting this and allowing it to settle in your mind that this issue/problem must be released without any further thoughts about it and cross it off your list.

Every day this next week be aware and notice when you are stressing, also notice which activities bring about stress. Every night before bed write down what is on your mind that's bothering you or what bothered you throughout the day. It's a great idea to keep a stress journal as then you'll be able to see patterns, addressing the issues that you don't feel deserve the amount of stress that it's causing you and it will be easier to manage it. Notice what things seem to make you nervous and keep writing things down on a daily basis, spending time analyzing what the root cause of the stress for you is. Often times writing things down in a very clear and logical way helps to see a solution or otherwise brings about clarity about how insignificant the issue truly is.

Remember that doing this exercise 'in your head' defeats the purpose. Writing it all out and allowing enough time each day to do this without a rush is vital. Commit to the process.

FORTH WEEK: Declutter your life

The simpler life is, the better and you can't live a simple life when your house is cluttered with things, especially things you don't need or use. It's time to go through your house, each and every room and give away or throw away items that you truly don't need. If you haven't used an item I over 6 months and the item doesn't serve any real purpose, isn't sentimental and doesn't bring you joy then it should go. This will feel like a cleansing of sorts and also if you're giving the items away to someone who needs them it serves as a double purpose. Also make a commitment to buy less, choose not to be a consumer but instead always ask yourself whether you really need this item or whether it's the addiction speaking. Make a habit to not give material possessions as gifts and instead think of gifts you can make or activities you can do together.

STEP SIX

Fill with positive

When we are very young children we truly love ourselves. We don't think we are too fat, too poor, too slow, too loud and self judgement or critical thinking doesn't exist. Things are very simple and we are honest about what we want, we do what makes us happy and it's easy to have fun no matter the circumstances. As we grow into adults we are molded by society, we learn about what's right and wrong, what's expected of us and we learn that there are levels of beauty, levels of class, levels of intelligence. We learn to judge one another, judge ourselves and constantly compare us to the next person. We get so caught up in our goals, needs, wishes and being perfect that we lose all sense of self. We try so hard to be the best employee, get perfect grades, be the perfect spouse, to not be ordinary, to be the best parent and our world revolves around pleasing others and fulfilling this ego of what we wish we were. We try so hard to excel in our job or career, convincing ourselves that this is absolutely the most vital and important thing in life becoming totally consumed with being the best in our field, the top, the most successful, the most rewarded and acknowledged. A lifetime is spent to make more money, get more security, achieve more financial freedom, save more, get the promotion although nobody would say that work means more to them than family, more than health, more than love and yet from everyone's actions it seems that work must be the most important thing in the world. It's this total imbalance and disconnect that causes strain and misery. Eventually we lose our freedom to be ourselves, we forget what's important, we become very self critical and we get so caught up in living life to others expectations or the high standards we set up for ourselves that we forget the simple yet utterly important element that children possess... to just have fun. Of course work is important and so is school, being a good parent or doing well in whatever project you're working on but it's vital to be honest enough with ourselves and put this in perspective with everything else that's important and have the ability to dedicate our time, effort and energy accordingly to the things that matter. So if work is 6th on your priority list then make sure you don't spend 90% of your energies on work as that's a clear imbalance. Performing, succeeding, earning becomes an addiction just like crack cocaine so make sure you're not addicted to being something or reaching some place. As the Dalai Lama said 'The interesting thing about greed is that although the underlying motive is to seek satisfaction, even after obtaining what you want, you're still not satisfied. It's this endless, nagging desire for more that leads to trouble. On the other hand, if you're truly contented, it doesn't matter whether you get what you want or not. Either way, you remain content.' It's alright to achieve something or earn something but this shouldn't be something you cannot live without. It's important to wake up and see this madness for what it is and find balance and simplicity in your life, accepting that at some point you have enough. More and more people are finding that having and living a simple life is the answer. Having less material possessions, less responsibility, less chores, working only as much as you have to and spending time doing the things that are actually enjoyable and truly important to you is what will bring you satisfaction and happiness.

Don't be defined by ONE thing

Being consumed with one thing in life is unhealthy and usually ends in misery. Maybe you focus all your energy on being a parent or a career path but remember whatever you are or whatever you are trying to be shouldn't define you. Putting too much emphasis on one thing builds huge pressure for it to fully complete you and if you lose that one thing then you are crushed. There should not be a job, a person or a project that you cannot live without or that you desperately need. Maybe you're thinking that you need to be that focussed to succeed or that you don't have time for anything else besides that one thing you spend all your time on but this is just not a healthy way to spend your life. I'm not suggesting you don't care about your work or passions, I'm simply suggesting to find balance and fill you life with numerous enjoyable activities, relationships, projects and purpose that isn't single themed. And if you feel that you don't have time for other things besides your career or besides being a parent or besides school then you need to change something, shift something around, to achieve better time management. How can you change your life around so that it doesn't put this pressure on you and so you have no time for anything except work? Or if you spend all your time taking care of kids then figure out a way to work out a plan to make space for other things. There is always a way if you truly want to find one. You need to have time to enjoy life without just thinking that you'll enjoy life eventually, on the weekend, next month, on that vacation or when you retire. Life is about enjoying it now so if you don't have the time to do things you love then it's time to change it up.

Enjoy the simple things

Another trick to leading a more positive life is not so much doing more fun things as learning to have fun doing the things you find tedious or boring. You know when you watch a movie and there is that feel good montage where the character is cleaning the house or doing some other regular thing but they are listening to music, dancing around and enjoying it? Well you should try that too! Don't only look forward to those once a month events while hating the rest of your time. Instead dance while you mop the floor and sing really loud when you do the dishes. Play your favorite album, play games, chase your loved one around the house, let go, be more easy going and try to find that innocence you had as a child. I want you to try make this a daily goal, to try to enjoy every single moment as much as possible throughout the day. So from waking up, try to lay in bed for a couple of minutes and really enjoy waking up, stretch, give yourself a head rub, smile, giggle, wiggle your toes, put on your favorite music... brush your teeth while wiggling your hips, make funny faces into the mirror, take some deep breaths and imagine what wonderful things you wish to happen today. Appreciate the food you eat for breakfast and enjoy every last bite, even if you're eating the most mundane and ordinary thing. When driving, practice smiling the whole time and listen to your favorite music. When you pass people whether it's someone you know or a total stranger take the time to smile at them and say 'good morning' or a 'hello' and really look at them, make eye contact, we all need more eye contact, and hugs! We all need more hugs! Hug your partner every morning and hug them throughout the day, hug your kids, hug your dog, hug your store attendant, hug anyone you can! Hugs produce oxytocin in the brain that gives you the 'feel good' energy. Imagine someone was filming you the entire time throughout the day, how would you look? Would you be going through the day with a frown on your face, just waiting for it to be over and rushing like mad to get everything done? Or can you instill some joy and peace into your surroundings, spread some good will to others and inspire others to smile?

Love yourself

Do you truly love yourself? Some think this is somehow egotistical or selfish but I think it's important to be in love with yourself. This doesn't mean you walk around putting others down or being big headed, it just means that you love spending time with yourself, you are comfortable with who you are and you love everything about yourself. You shouldn't judge yourself, you shouldn't speak or think unkindly about yourself, you don't need to beat yourself down. It means you know who you are, you believe in yourself, you would want to be friends with someone who was like you and that you genuinely think you are a good person. If you do have some issues with yourself or points that you feel uncomfortable with then it's time to look at that and ask how you can improve on those aspects of your character? If you are not happy with you then how can others around you be? And instead of seeing all the little physical flaws and things you'd like to change or wish that were different, rather see how perfectly beautiful you are! Accept all the parts of you and know that this body is just a vessel, it's not you defined, it's just a shell and the more you love your body and accept it, the more the real you, inside, will feel incredible. When you see someone who feels good about themselves it doesn't matter what they're wearing or how skinny they are, it's their energy and their confidence that lights others up.

How often do you spoil yourself? I want you to really think back and ask yourself when was the last time you spoiled yourself? Not your kids or partner or friend… but you, and you alone? Just like you spoil a loved one on a special occasion, why not take the time to spoil yourself? Why not plan a date with yourself? Whether you're single or not this should be done without waiting to meet "the one" who will spoil you and without putting that pressure on your partner if you have one, to spoil you, but to simply spoil yourself. Loving yourself and showing that love to yourself is the first step and it's a vital one.

Meditation

Meditation comes in many different forms and I believe this to be the answer for many issues people carry around. It has been used for thousands of years all over the world and although some use chanting meditations and some are silent, some use music or sounds and some are in groups and some alone, they all pretty much use the same basic principle which is to quieten your mind and to focus on the breath while feeling the sensations in your body. For someone who has never tried meditation before, they can begin with just 5 minute sessions each day or if you can start off with a longer session of 10 or 15 minutes that's even better. Anyone, no matter how scattered they are, should be able to have the will power to sit still for five minutes a day.

It's best to meditate upon waking up but if you cannot do it in the morning then any time of the day will do. It's best to practice in a place that's as quiet as possible with few distractions but if you cannot find a quiet place then use some ear plugs. Sit on the floor so you feel grounded unless you cannot do this due to physical limitations, then you can sit on a chair. Choose a place where disturbances will be low and definitely turn off your cellphone. It's best to have a place in the house where children or others won't be running through and best to have a small space set aside for meditation that's not used for anything else. Some people enjoy making it a ceremony and it helps them to have a special mat to sit on, light incense or candles but it's all optional, you could just as easily meditate sitting on the floor in the corner of your bedroom. Sit either cross legged or whatever other comfortable position you want, know that no matter what position you sit in, it will start to become uncomfortable eventually but try to avoid moving around and really focus on being completely still. Close your eyes and keep them closed the entire time. Try not to scratch, itch, check things and really focus on clearing your mind and focusing on the breath. Every time you notice yourself thinking, don't judge yourself but simply bring your focus back to your breath. Try not to control your breath, just notice it coming in and out and try to keep the mind clear. The purpose of the exercise is to sit in complete stillness for whatever time you committed to and to constantly be aware if any thoughts come into the mind, when they do simply stopping them and bringing your attention back to your breath. This is such a simple exercise but so hard although the more you practice it, the better you'll get. Start with just five minutes if it's really difficult and work your way up. So after the first week of doing it, move it up to 6 minutes next week and then up to 8 and then 10 and eventually hopefully you can sit for up to an hour. You'll start to notice how your entire demeanor changes towards people, circumstances and the world in general. Research shows that meditating regularly does so much for the physical and mental state such as eliminating anxiety, strengthening self esteem, lowering stress levels and regulating hormones. You'll suddenly have more patience with things that drove you nuts before and you'll feel more peaceful. If you give it a real try for 30 days you will notice huge benefits.

* * *

THE EXERCISE:

* Meditation: Commit to trying meditation for 30 days. Even if it's only for 5 minutes a day that you sit in silence and stillness but try to do it for longer as the days go on. Make a note on your calendar when you start and write down the amount of time you have meditated each day so you can keep track it. Do not meditate for less time as the days go on but make sure you are meditating for more time each week. Ultimately by the last week I hope you can sit for at least 30 minutes every day. I sincerely hope you can make meditation part of your life for good long after the exercise is over.

* Priority list: Write down your top five priorities, most important at the top. Really spend time thinking about this, imagine if you lost your health, your car, your family, your loved one, your home, your job.... which ones are most important? Now make a list of the top five things you spend the most time thinking/worrying about with the one you spend the most time on at the top. Compare the two lists. Is the thing you think most about in the top five on your list? If not then think about how you can put this into perspective and see that might not deserve all your time and that you should put effort into other things that are more important to you. Put your priority list up somewhere you can see it every day so you don't lose sight of what's important.

* Hobbies: I want you to make a list of ten things that you truly love to do. They can be outdoor activities, dancing lessons, reading a great novel, gardening or whatever you like, but be specific and avoid using phrases like 'spend time with friends'. Once you make the list, make sure you include those things at least three times a week. If you need to add it to your schedule then do so but don't push this aside or forget about it. Do not let an entire week pass by without doing something you enjoy. Make a commitment that at the very minimum once a week, but hopefully you can commit to three or four times a week. Also once in a while truly go out of your way and plan something really special for yourself. Something that you don't do often or maybe something you wish someone else would plan or do for you. Spoil yourself and actually enjoy spending time with yourself as if you were your own best friend.

* Try dedicate an entire week to this exercise. From when you wake up until you go to sleep, attempt to enjoy every single thing you do no matter what it is. Ask yourself how you can make everything more enjoyable and truly practice this throughout the day. Every time you are about to do a chore or an activity, take a second to think about how you can make it more fun. If you can do this even a little on a daily basis, it will make life much much more enjoyable.

* This is another week long exercise and it's also the last! I want you to spend time being actively kind to others. Each day upon waking, make a commitment that you will treat every person you come across as if they were a loved one

or family member and take the time to really say hello to them, make eye contact, give them a compliment or show kindness. Each time someone speaks to you, not just your best friend but the gardener, the guy working at the post office, the waitress, anyone, stop whatever you're doing and engage with them, listen to them and be genuinely interested. Also each and every day do something kind for someone. A good deed or a favor. If you can start giving more then you will start receiving more as this is the rule of the universe.

CONCLUSION

You made it!

Well done, you made it to the end! It's now time to thank yourself and be proud. I hope you really utilized these steps and that they helped you. Remember that lasting change shouldn't stop when you stop reading and I want you to stick to everything that we tried to implement throughout this book. Hopefully you are more aware in all areas of life and it will be easier to pin point where the issues are stemming from in the future. Make sure you don't live out of balance and be healthy physically as well as mentally. Remember that nobody is perfect and we all take two steps forward and one step back but don't give up and know that as long as you are trying that's what will get you there. Take care of yourself, love yourself, forgive yourself. Allow yourself to be the person you were born to be. Remember you were not born to be angry, overworked, stressed, negative, tired, sick or jealous. Let the beautiful qualities flourish and allow the bad ones to melt away. Take care of what you eat and rid yourself of addictions of all kind. All things are alright in moderation and as long as you are doing the best you can that's good enough. Keep pushing, keep trying, keep laughing and keep loving. Love everyone around you not just those close to you or family members as if we all looked out for one another, strangers included, the world would be a better place.

Thank you for taking this journey with me. I sincerely hope that you were able to learn something from my book. I hope you committed 100% to the process and if you ever find yourself lost again I hope you return to this book and maybe try it all over again. If you can keep it up, it will become easier and more natural to stay positive, eat healthy and avoid the bad stuff (physically and mentally speaking) as the hardest part is the beginning, the hardest part is to take the steps to change yourself but the rest just gets easier as time goes on. It's not easy but it's definitely worth it as nothing is more important than being healthy and happy for as long as you are here.

RECIPES:

NATURAL MOUTH WASH

* 4 cups water

* 1/2 tsp tea tree oil

This is antibacterial and makes your breath smell wonderful! I would never put chemical laden liquids in my mouth. I use an old jar or little bottle that I keep in my bathroom and re-fill as needed. Adjust the strength of the tea tree, if you like it stronger then add more, if it's too strong then add less.

COCONUT OIL

Coconut oil is a great substitute for many toxic toiletries and can be used for many uses such as face moisturizer, body moisturizer, hair leave in conditioner, make up remover, diaper cream, prevent stretch marks, natural spf5 sunscreen or mixed with sugar to use as a body scrub,

NATURAL TOOTHPASTE

* 5 tbsp baking soda

* 5 tbsp coconut oil

* 1 tbsp water

* 10 - 30 drops of essential oil, depending on how strong you want the flavor (peppermint, eucalyptus, spearmint, tea tree or anything else!)

Simple, cheap and does the body good. Mix all the ingredients into a paste, spoon into a small glass jar or container and use a dab every time you brush your teeth.

LIQUID DISH SOAP

* 5 cups boiling water

* 4 Tbsp borax

* 4 Tbsp grated bar soap (use castile bar soap, Ivory, or whichever natural bar you prefer)

* 30 - 40 drops essential oils, optional (find 100% pure essential oils here)

There are many great natural dish soaps now in stores but if you want to make your own then here is a good one!

Boil water. Combine borax and grated bar soap in a medium bowl. Pour hot water over the mixture. Whisk until the grated soap is completely melted. Allow mixture to cool on the counter top for 6-8 hours, stirring occasionally. Dish soap will gel upon standing.

Transfer to a squirt bottle, and add essential oils (if using). Shake well to combine. Store the left over in a container.

LIQUID HAND WASH

* Fill bottle with 1/3 of Bronner's soap.

* Add 5 drops of essential oil of your choice (lavender, eucalyptus, mint, tea tree oil)

* Fill the rest with water

Purchase a large bottle of the Bronner's Castile Liquid Soap. It's all natural without any toxic chemicals. You can actually use it instead of soap for your body too! Also get a hand soap dispenser bottle with a pump and in it you can make your own mix of liquid hand soap.

VINEGAR CLEANING SOLUTION

Vinegar cleans like an all-purpose cleaner and all you need to do is mix an equal part of vinegar and water in a spray bottle and then you have a solution that will clean most areas of your home. Don't worry about the smell as it vanishes once the solution dries! Vinegar is a great natural cleaning product as well as a disinfectant and deodorizer and remember that you should always test any cleaning solution on a small area first to make sure it's not damaging or removing color. Improperly diluted vinegar solution will be too acidic and can strip certain colors and it shouldn't be used on marble surfaces either. You can use this solution to clean your bathroom including the tub, toilet, sinks and mop the floor with it as well as the kitchen and other rooms.

LEMON JUICE CLEANING SOLUTION

Lemon juice is great for shinning any metal surfaces such as copper or brass as well as cleaning any tough soap scum. You can mix lemon juice with either baking soda or vinegar to increase the cleaning power.

BAKING SODA AS A DEODORIZER

Baking soda can be used to clean pretty much anything but it also works as a deodorizer anywhere you have unwanted smells. You can sprinkle it in smelly shoes, put an opened box in your fridge or trash cans and laundry. It's an essential cleaning agent as good as any you will purchase in the store and it's natural!

FURNITURE POLISH

* 1 cup olive oil

* 1/2 cup lemon juice

Mix and use on your hardwood furniture to give you a beautiful polish!

CARPET STAIN REMOVER

* 1 cup hydrogen peroxide

* 1 cup water

* 1 Tbsp baking soda

Random stain spots, red wine, pet urine or any other carpet stains will be gone with this! Put following ingredients in a spray bottle. Shake up and spray onto stains, wait until dry and go again on any more spots. (I would test it on a small piece of carpet first and if it bleaches it out at all then lessen the amount of hydrogen peroxide you put in).

NATURAL BLEACH ALTERNATIVE

* 6 cups water

* 1/4 cup lemon juice

* 1/2 hydrogen peroxide*

Use this to soak your items in or just add to your laundry. Can also be used to bleach bathroom or other surface places. Mix all the ingredients together and add 2 cups per wash load or put in spray bottle and use as a household cleaner.

LAUNDRY DETERGENT

* 1 bar (or 4.5 ounces) of shaved bar soap (Dr. Bronner's, Ivory, ZOTE)*

* 1 cup borax*

* 1 cup of washing soda*

Mix thoroughly for 5 minutes and use! You can add this to your blender or processor to make a fine powder to use in even cold water laundry loads. Store in a small sealed contained and use small scoop for every load. Should be enough for 32 - 50 loads.

DISINFECTANT SPRAY

* 1 cup water*

* 10 drops lavender essential oil*

* 10 drops thyme or eucalyptus oil*

* 5 drops tea tree oil*

This has all the antibiotic, antibacterial, antiviral and anti fungal properties without any of the harmful chemicals. Mix all ingredients in a spray bottle and use on any hard surface around your home.

NATURAL GLASS CLEANER

* 1/4 cup rubbing alcohol

* 1/4 cup white vinegar

* 1 tbsp corn starch

* 2 cups distilled or boiled water

If the bottle tells you to wear gloves then it's probably not something you should spray anywhere inside or even near your home. Here is a solution for cleaning glass. Combine everything in a spray bottle and shake well. Also shake before each use as corn starch will settle on the bottom.

FABRIC SOFTENER

* 3 cups warm water

* 1.5 cups white vinegar

* 1 cup natural hair conditioner (optional for extra softness)

* essential oil for the smell (optional)

Pour all ingredients into a large container and stir. Add 1/4 cup per load. I personally don't use any fabric softener as I see this as an extra luxury that I don't really need but if you do use fabric softeners know that most are super toxic, staying in your clothing long after the wash, leeching into your skin so it's best to use something natural if you must soften your fabrics.

Connect with Arunya Villiers

Website: www.ArunyaVilliers.com

Email: arunya@arunyavilliers.com

Facebook: www.Facebook.com/arunyavilliers

ARUNYA VILLIERS

6 STEPS TO HEALTH & HAPPINESS

www.ingramcontent.com/pod-product-compliance
Lightning Source LLC
Chambersburg PA
CBHW022254290526
45785CB00015B/770